Public Health Approaches to Health Promotion

Healthy behaviors, at the individual and community levels, are imperative to improving and sustaining better public health. With a strong focus on prevention, health promotion strategies are crucial to improving quality of life, while taking into account the various determinants of health. This book provides a global perspective, with an emphasis on contextual issues with health promotion in South Asia for understanding challenges and related strategies. Readers will be comprehensively introduced to healthy behaviors through case studies, covering theories, interventions, and approaches to promote healthy behavior, the impact of policy, and how behavior change can be sustained.

Key features

- Covers existing and emerging issues in health promotion
- Input from globally renowned public health experts with a multidisciplinary approach to content and audience
- Connects with health systems and relevant sustainable development goals
- Provides case studies for enabling readers to understand and apply evidence-based solutions to key public health issues

Public Health Approach

Public Health Approach to Cardiovascular Disease Prevention & Management
Edited by Dorairaj Prabhakaran, Shuchi Anand, and K. Srinath Reddy

Public Health Approaches to Health Promotion
Monika Arora and Shifalika Goenka

Public Health Approaches to Health Promotion

Edited by
Monika Arora and Shifalika Goenka

CRC Press
Taylor & Francis Group
Boca Raton London New York

CRC Press is an imprint of the
Taylor & Francis Group, an **informa** business

Designed cover image: Shutterstock

First edition published 2024
by CRC Press
6000 Broken Sound Parkway NW, Suite 300, Boca Raton, FL 33487-2742

and by CRC Press
4 Park Square, Milton Park, Abingdon, Oxon, OX14 4RN

CRC Press is an imprint of Taylor & Francis Group, LLC

ISBN: 9781032571751 (hbk)
ISBN: 9781138592681 (pbk)
ISBN: 9781003438182 (ebk)

DOI: 10.1201/b23385

Typeset in Palatino
by Deanta Global Publishing Services, Chennai, India

Dedicated to the millions of marginalized people living in lower- and middle-income countries (LMICs), including India. We hope that the content of the book will inspire the thought processes and actions of students and health professionals throughout the world.

Table of Contents

Preface

The first International Conference on Health Promotion was conducted in Ottawa, Canada, in 1986, which went on to change the drift of various public health actions. Health promotion, defined as "the process of enabling people to increase control over, and to improve their health," has ever since evolved and is now acknowledged as a broad umbrella that aims to provide an individual with all the resources to enable a healthy decision-making process to promote their health and general well-being. Health promotion accounts for the fact that health outcomes are encompassed within a spectrum of social, economic, and political forces, and that biomedical interventions alone cannot suffice in the long run if we are to aim for a healthier nation and a healthier world.

The last few decades have seen a drastic increase in the prevalence of noncommunicable diseases (NCDs), with the top three causes of mortality being strongly attributed to lifestyle choices. This is alongside the unfinished agenda of communicable diseases and newly emerging diseases. While the prevalence of diseases such as cancers, cardiovascular conditions, and respiratory disorders continue to rise, many low- and middle-income countries (LMICs) continue to grapple with the dual burden of NCDs as well as communicable diseases brought upon due to lack of access to safe food, water, and environment. A vast spectrum of risk factors impact behavioral choices, ranging from unsafe food and water to several commercial determinants of health. On one hand, technological and digital advances have benefited health innovations, but on the other hand, they have posed new risk factors due to excessive interaction with social media leading to easy access to misinformation and unregulated content, lack of physical activity, increased screen exposure, and exposure to unhealthy product advertisements.

This book was created with the intent to compile a comprehensive resource that addresses the long-standing challenges in public health, especially in LMICs, as well as provide evidence-based contemporary health promotion solutions to these problems. *Public Health Approaches to Health Promotion* provides a practical guide to students and practitioners to apply principles of health promotion to address social, political, environmental, and related barriers to enable the adoption of healthy behaviors at the individual, family, community, and at the population level; and sustain this behavior change with supportive policy interventions. The book places special emphasis on the interconnectedness of the health domain with social, economic, geographical determinants, and with development agenda; and underscores the need for adoption of a multisectoral and a whole-of-society approach, citing successful models and case studies from an LMIC perspective. Case studies and examples have been selected to help students and practitioners to understand processes to follow in designing multisectoral, multicomponent, and interdisciplinary interventions for promoting health.

The book is largely led by authors from low- and middle-income countries who have personally designed, implemented, or evaluated several health promotion programs and policies. Many earlier books on health promotion have largely explained theories and frameworks based on experiences and in the context of developed countries. This book highlights the challenges of LMICs and how health promotion interventions and programs have been adapted to local contexts leading to success. This volume envisages that readers enjoy and learn practical applications of models and theories of health promotion.

About the Editors

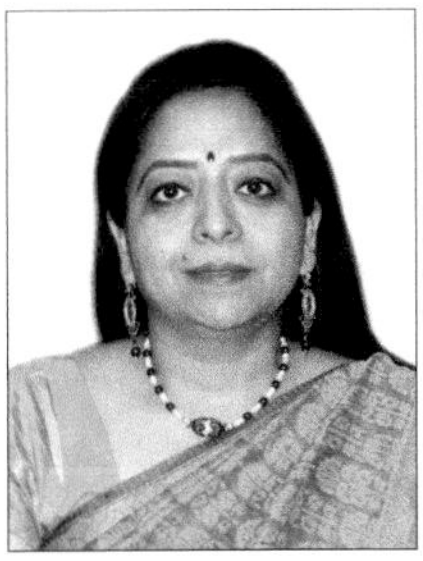

Monika Arora is a public health scientist working in the area of preventing and managing noncommunicable diseases (NCDs) through health promotion and health advocacy. She is a Vice President (Research and Health Promotion) at the Public Health Foundation of India and has a special interest in NCD policy research, health impact assessment (HIA), and program evaluations. She is Executive Director of HRIDAY (Health Related Information Dissemination Amongst Youth), an NGO working on NCD prevention and control, and youth and patient engagement; and hosts the secretariat for Healthy India Alliance (India NCD Alliance). She has served as president-elect of the NCD Alliance (2021–2023) and chairperson of the South East Asia NCD Alliance (2020–2023).

She has published extensively in the area of preventing NCD risk factors in different health promotion settings, particularly in the area of multisectoral action for NCD prevention and control. She has actively contributed to closing the research gap, and her research outcomes have successfully informed policies, training, and programs at national and regional levels. Arora has been a member of various national and international expert committees on NCD-related policies and programs, including an expert committee formed by the World Health Organization Director General on ending childhood obesity.

Arora was honored with the Best Practices Award in Global Health in 2011 by the Global Health Council for demonstrating best practice examples in the area of preventing NCDs among youth in community settings. She was also awarded the WHO Director General's World No Tobacco Day Award in 2012, the Exceptional Women of Excellence 2018 Award by the Women Economic Forum (WEF) in April 2018, the Dr. Prem Menon Outstanding Service Award in January 2018 by the World-India Diabetes Foundation (WIDF) in recognition of her contributions to the education and prevention of diabetes among children in India and "SAHM 2023 International Chapter Award - Northern Hemisphere" by Society for Adolescent Health and Medicine (SAHM).

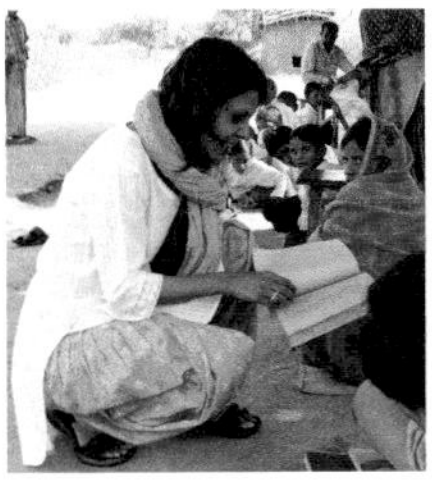

Shifalika Goenka is a physician and public health professional as well as a Professor and Director-Bioethics at the Public Health Foundation of India. She also heads the Health Promotion and Physical Activity program at the Centre for Chronic Disease Control (CCDC), a WHO Collaborating Centre for Surveillance Capacity Building & Translational Research in cardiometabolic Diseases. She has led the health promotion component of one of the largest worksite projects in India for the prevention of noncommunicable diseases and obesity. The World Economic Forum recognised this program as the 'best practice'. She was Commissioner and regional representative on the Lancet Commission on Obesity (which got a lot of media publicity as the Syndemic Commission). She was also a co-author on the Lancet Series on Physical Activity and Public Health. She led the Indian adaptation and validation of the first international physical activity measurement instrument and is the country representative on the Global Report Card on physical activity. Her areas of interest have expanded to the built environment and transport systems and their powerful role in enhancing physical activity in populations, and lowering carbon emissions, decreasing accidents, and the role of green spaces.

She strongly believes that providing a health-promoting nutritional, physical and social environment, to each and every human being, forms the foundations of health promotion. How can an individual who doesn't know where his next meal will come from, who does not have water in his taps, or clean drinking water to drink, or a roof over his head or a park which he can go to, and whose children can't go to school, how is he expected to decide and take control of having more fruits and vegetables in his diet or exercising?

List of Contributors

Ritvik Amarchand
Scientist-D, Centre for Community Medicine, All India Institute of Medical Sciences (AIIMS), India

Atul Ambekar
Professor, National Drug Dependence Treatment Centre and Department of Psychiatry, All India Institute of Medical Sciences, India

Monika Arora
Vice President (Research and Health Promotion)
Public Health Foundation of India

Upendra Bhojani
Director and the DBT/Wellcome Trust India Alliance Fellow, Institute of Public Health, Bangalore; and University of Durham, United Kingdom

Himanshu Burte
Associate Professor, Centre for Urban Science and Engineering (CUSE), Indian Institute of Technology (IIT-B), Powai, Mumbai

Mansi Chopra
Senior Research Scientist, HRIDAY, New Delhi

Aastha Chugh
Research Scientist, HRIDAY, New Delhi

Neha Dahiya
Senior Resident, Department of Community Medicine & School of Public Health, PGIMER, Chandigarh, India

Preet K. Dhillon
Public Health Foundation of India, Gurugram, India; and Centre for Chronic Disease Control, New Delhi, India

Chetna Duggal
Associate Professor, Tata Institute of Social Sciences, Mumbai, India

Mona Duggal
Assistant Professor, Community Advanced Eye Centre, PGIMER, Chandigarh; and Adjunct professor, IIIT, Delhi, India

Shifalika Goenka
Head, Health Promotion and Physical Activity, Centre for Chronic Disease Control (CCDC) | WHO Collaborating Center for Surveillance Capacity Building, and Translational Research in Cardio-metabolic Diseases, Delhi, India
Director-Bioethics, Public Health Foundation of India

Aprajita Gogoi
Executive Director, Centre for Catalyzing Change, Delhi, India

Ayon Gupta
Centre for Community Medicine, All India Institute of Medical Sciences (AIIMS), New Delhi, India

Melissa Blythe Harrell
Professor, University of Texas Health Science Center at Houston, Texas

Gregory W. Heath
Guerry Professor Emeritus in Public Health, University of Tennessee at Chattanooga; and Epidemiologist and Adjunct Professor of Medicine, University of Tennessee Health Science Center College of Medicine, Chattanooga, Tennessee

Pragati Hebbar
PhD Scholar and DBT/Wellcome Trust India Alliance Early Career Fellow and Assistant Director, Institute of Public Health, Bengaluru, India

Vikram Jha
Advisor and Consultant, Medical Education and Health Care, India

Neeru S. Juneja
Founder, Udyam Trust, New Delhi, India

Thejas Kathrikolly
Research Scholar, Department of Community Medicine, Kasturba Medical College, Manipal Academy of Higher Education (MAHE), Manipal, India

Sonali Khan
Managing Director, Sesame Workshop India, Delhi, India

Shweta Khandelwal
Head, Nutrition Research, and additional professor, Public Health Foundation of India, Gurugram, India

Asha Kilaru
RMNCH Consultant; and Co-founder, Bangalore Birth Network, India

Anand Krishnan
Professor, Centre for Community Medicine, All India Institute of Medical Sciences (AIIMS), India

Malini Krishnankutty
Centre for Urban Science and Engineering (CUSE), Indian Institute of Technology (IIT-B), Powai, Mumbai

Muralidhar M. Kulkarni
Associate Professor, Department of Community Medicine, Kasturba Medical College, Manipal, Manipal Academy of Higher Education, Udupi District, Karnataka

Glenn Laverack
Adjunct Full Professor, College of Medicine & Health Sciences, Institute of Public Health, UAE University, Al Ain, United Arab Emirates

Ravi Mehrotra
Emory University, Rollins School of Public Health, Atlanta, Georgia

G.K. Mini
Associate Professor, Global Institute of Public Health, Ananthapuri Hospitals and Research Institute, Kerala, India

Gauravi A. Mishra
Professor and Physician, Department of Preventive Oncology, Centre for Cancer Epidemiology, Homi Bhabha National Institute, Tata Memorial Centre, Mumbai, India

Dinesh Mohan
Honorary Professor, Indian Institute of Technology, Delhi, India

Vikrant Mohanty
Maulana Azad Institute of Dental Sciences, New Delhi, India

Suma Nair
Professor and Head, Community Medicine; and Coordinator, Centre for Community Oncology, Kasturba Medical College, Manipal, Manipal Academy of Higher Education (MAHE)

Mark Parascandola
Director, Research and Training Branch, Center for Global Health, National Cancer Institute, Bethesda, Maryland, USA

Tulsi Patel
Professor of Sociology, Delhi School of Economics, University of Delhi, Delhi, India

Sanjay Patnaik
Indian Institute of Public Health, Delhi, India

David Patterson
Global Health Law Groningen Research Centre, Faculty of Law, University of Groningen, Netherlands; and Member, Steering Group, EUPHA Law and Public Health Section

Sharmila A. Pimple
Professor and Physician, Department of Preventive Oncology, Tata Memorial Hospital, Mumbai, India

Nupur Prakash
Gender and Law Analyst at IDLO - International Development Law Organization, India

Suneet Singh Puri
Research Associate, Darpana Academy of Performing Arts, Ahmedabad, India

Jayasree Ramachandran
Research Scholar, Department of Community Medicine, Kasturba Medical College, Manipal Academy of Higher Education (MAHE), Manipal, India

Chythra R. Rao
Associate Professor, Kasturba Medical College Manipal, Manipal, India

Eram Rao
Professor, Department of Food Technology, Bhaskaracharya College of Applied Sciences, University of Delhi, India

Tina Rawal
Research Scientist, Health Promotion Division, Public Health Foundation of India

Sunetra Roday
Senior Advisor, Content and Special Projects, Food Future Foundation, New Delhi
and
Former Principal
Maharashtra State Institute of Hotel Management and Catering Technology, Pune

Sunanda K. Reddy
Chairperson (Honorary), CARENIDHI Trust, New Delhi, India

Syamant Sandhir
Director, customer experience, Futurescape, Gurugram, India

Mallika Sarabhai
Co-Director, Darpana Academy of Performing Arts, Ahmedabad, India

Gina Sharma
Office of the president and head, External Communications and Digital Media, Public Health Foundation of India

Ranjitha S. Shetty
Associate Professor, Kasturba Medical College Manipal, Manipal, India

Krithiga Shridhar
Senior Research Scientist and Associate Professor (adjunct), Centre for Chronic Conditions and Injuries, Public Health Foundation of India

Surbhi Shrivastava
PhD candidate, Department of Sociology, Emory University, Atlanta, Georgia

Archana Singh
Additional Professor, Biochemistry, AIIMS New Delhi

Shalini Singh
Assistant Professor, National Drug Dependence Treatment Centre, All India Institute of Medical Sciences, New Delhi, India

Navsharan Singh
Senior Programme Specialist, Social and Economic Policy International Development Research Centre | Centre de recherches pour le développement international, Asia Regional Office, New Delhi, India

Pubudu Sumanasekara
Alcohol and Drug Information Centre, Colombo, Sri Lanka

Venkata Ratnadeep Suri
Assistant Professor, SSH, IIIT-Delhi, India

K.R. Thankappan
Professor, Department of Public Health and Community Medicine, Central University Kerala

Geetam Tiwari
Professor, Civil Engineering Department, Indian Institute of Technology, Delhi

Ian Warwick
Associate Professor, Department of Education, Policy and Practice IOE, UCL's Faculty of Education and Society, London, UK

Paula Wheeler
Equitable place-based health and care theme manager and neighborhood coordinator, NIHR ARC North West Coast, Lancaster University, England

Reviewers

Mark Parascandola, Chief, Research and Training Branch Center for Global Health, National Cancer Institute, Bethesda, Maryland

Ian Warwick, Associate professor and program leader, Institute of Education, University College London, England

Glenn Laverack, Visiting professor, Department of Sociology and Social Research, University of Trento, Italy

TECHNICAL SUPPORT TEAM

Tina Rawal, Research scientist, Public Health Foundation of India

Neha Jain, Research fellow, Public Health Foundation of India

SECTION I

HEALTH PROMOTION APPROACHES

A Perspective: Promoting Health and Well-Being through Values-Based Practice

Ian Warwick

As outlined in Chapter 1, there are a number of key issues to keep in mind when adopting a 'health promotion imagination'. These include understanding health and well-being (or disease and ill health) as influenced by factors operating at and across micro, meso, and macro levels.

Through its strategies and action areas, the Ottawa Charter begins to identify what sorts of activities at which sorts of levels might build on people's needs, concerns, interests, and strengths to help reduce illness and enhance a sense of well-being. Yet perhaps underplayed in health promotion overall are the values that might inform professionals working to promote health, via research, practice, or policy.

In this short reflective piece, I draw from well-being–related research carried out with colleagues at the Institute of Education in London.[1] I suggest that, while not unimportant, research 'evidence' should be viewed skeptically and that rather than being 'evidence-based', professional practice in health promotion should be values-based. As it is only through placing values at the center of practice, can professionals respond and adapt to the continually changing and complex circumstances that shape and are shaped through people's lives.

Evidence-based practice (EBP), often initially associated with the Cochrane Collaboration's evidence-based medical initiatives in the early 1990s, has come to hold a certain appeal for some in education, nursing, social work, and health promotion. The calls to identify what works in this or that field of practice often rely on the simplification of social lives through their quantification and an assumed easy generalizability from one context to another. This rather removes our understanding of people's lives (and how best to respond to them) from the complexities of a layered nature of reality suggested by the Ottawa Charter (and its theoretical underpinnings related to social-ecological theory). However, notwithstanding its ongoing appeals to policymakers (McKnight and Morgan, 2020; Rogers, 2019), EBP has long been of concern to those working to support people's health and well-being (Mitchell, 1999; Tang et al., 2003; Biesta, 2010).

One key concern about adherence to EBP has been the removal of democratically oriented forms of professional practice (Biesta, 2010). While it may be possible to reduce the complexity of people's worlds – say, by having schools and other settings so tightly controlled that pupils and teachers have little or no say over ways of being and doing – it is certainly questionable as to whether this is desirable (Biesta, 2010).

Perhaps more useful for those working to promote health and well-being would be to discuss with one another what sorts of values should form the basis of my work. For example, the values underpinning health promotion have been said to focus on equity and a commitment to participatory practice as well as empowerment (Baum, 2021).

In our research on young people seeking asylum alone in the UK and on tackling homophobic bullying in secondary schools, we have drawn out five key values: working toward practical justice, a commitment to the sorts of research that promotes practical justice, adopting partnership-focused research, an orientation toward forms of inquiry that engage with multilayered realities of people's lives, and understanding the importance of temporality (how young people's needs, concerns, and interests can, and do, shift over time) (Aggleton et al., 2023).

Identifying the values that form the basis of health promotion can help us discuss and imagine ways of promoting health and well-being that are responsive to continuously changing contexts. Rather than prescribing professional practice, values-based health promotion allows for the emergence of new ways of thinking, being, and doing.

While I have outlined values that may prove useful (from Baum and my research), the point here is not to impose these but to encourage discussion about what, say, students in a school or members of the community consider important, relevant, and meaningful to their own and others' health and well-being.

NOTE

1. This research is described in more detail in Aggleton, Chase, and Warwick (under review).

DOI: 10.1201/b23385-2

REFERENCES

Aggleton, P., Chase, E. & Warwick, I., 2023. Young people, diversity, wellbeing and inclusion: towards values-led research and practice. Ch. 8 In C. Cameron, A. Koslowski, A, Lamont, and P. Moss (eds) *Social Research for our Times*. London: UCL Press.

Baum, F., 2021. Health promotion, health education, and the public's health. In Detels, R., Gulliford, M., Karim, Q.A. and Tan, C.C. eds., 2015. *Oxford Textbook of Global Public Health*. Oxford Textbook.

Biesta, G.J., 2010. Why 'what works' still won't work: From evidence-based education to value-based education. *Studies in Philosophy and Education*, *29*(5), pp. 491–503.

McKnight, L. and Morgan, A., 2020. A broken paradigm? What education needs to learn from evidence-based medicine. *Journal of Education Policy*, *35*(5), pp. 648–664.

Mitchell, G.J., 1999. Evidence-based practice: Critique and alternative view. *Nursing Science Quarterly*, *12*(1), pp. 30–35.

Rogers, B., 2019. Strengthening of the case for teacher judgement: A critique of the rationalities and technologies underpinning Gonski 2.0's renewed call for evidence-based practice. *Social Alternatives*, *38*(3), pp. 36–41.

Tang, K.C., Ehsani, J.P. and McQueen, D.V., 2003. Evidence based health promotion: Recollections, reflections, and reconsiderations. *Journal of Epidemiology & Community Health*, *57*(11), pp. 841–843.

1 Approaches to Health Promotion

Ayon Gupta, Ritvik Amarchand, and Anand Krishnan

CONTENTS

The greatest medicine of all is teaching people how not to need it.

Hippocrates of Kos

Health promotion is a holistic approach that moves beyond a focus on individual behavior toward a wider range of societal and environmental interventions and was defined in the Ottawa Charter on Health Promotion as the "process of enabling people to increase control over their health and its determinants, and thereby improve their health" (1). It involves three aspects: increasing awareness, providing skills, and creating a conducive environment to enable healthier choices. The Ottawa Charter incorporates five key action areas in health promotion (build healthy public policy, create supportive environments for health, strengthen community action for health, develop personal skills, and reorient health services) and three basic approaches (i.e., to enable, mediate, and advocate).

Health promotion is an integral part of public health as evident from the definition given by C.E.A. Winslow: "the science and art of preventing disease, prolonging life and promoting human health through organized efforts and informed choices of society, organizations, public and private, communities and individuals" (2). The 'new' public health requires a major shift toward a multilayered and holistic approach that empowers individuals and communities to take action for their own and others' health and well-being (3, 4). It should not only promote intersectoral action but also build ideas of health and well-being into public policies.

The main aim of healthy public policy is to create supportive environments that allow healthy choices to be readily accessible to citizens. A healthy public policy factors in health and equity considerations in all policy spheres. The Helsinki Declaration on Health in All Policies highlighted that health should be on the policy agenda in all sectors and at all government levels (5). An example of a healthy public policy is the MPOWER package for tobacco control, which includes the interventions of increasing taxes on tobacco products, instituting mandatory health warnings on tobacco products, and banning smoking in public spaces (6).

BOX 1.1 ANCIENT REFERENCES TO HEALTH PROMOTION

Ayurveda advocates lifestyle interventions. Some of these modalities are the concept of *Dinacharya* (daily health promotional activities), *Ritucharya* (health promotional activities during specific seasons), and *Aahara* (specific dietary regimens). Ayurveda views health as the outcome of the harmonized state of various elements: *Dosha*, *Dhatu*, *Mala*, and *Agni*.

A similar concept of harmony between the internal and external environment is also seen in the Greeks' apprehension of health and illness based on the theory of the four 'fluids' (blood, phlegm, yellow bile, and black bile). According to this tradition – mainly illustrated in Hippocrates's work *Air, Waters and Places* – health is defined based on an equilibrium achieved between environmental forces on the one hand (wind, temperature, water, ground, and food) and individual habits on the other (diet, alcohol, sexual behavior as well as work and leisure).

 DOI: 10.1201/b23385-3

EVOLUTION OF HEALTH PROMOTION CONCEPTS

Many ancient medical sciences used ideas consistent with the modern concept of health promotion (7, 8) (Box 1.1). In modern times, the term *primary prevention* was coined by Leavell and Clark and was used to describe "measures applicable to a particular disease or group of diseases to intercept the causes of disease before they involve man" (9). Though this definition was mostly disease-oriented, primary prevention included prevention of disease onset via risk reduction by altering behaviors or exposures that lead to disease or by enhancing resistance to the effects of exposure to a disease agent. Ever since the publication of the Lalonde Report in 1974 (10) by the Canadian government, there has been a growing recognition that the conventional 'biomedical' model is insufficient to address all health determinants. The Alma-Ata Declaration in 1978 emphasized the adoption of the principles of intersectoral coordination and equitable distribution on the road to 'health for all'. The focus of health promotion efforts thus changed from an emphasis on the individual to more structural factors in society that support the types of choices that people ultimately make. "Achieving Health for All: A Framework for Health Promotion", released in November 1986 (11), further developed the concept of health promotion, suggesting three strategies for increasing health promotion: fostering public participation, strengthening community health services, and healthy public policy. Figure 1.1 captures the progress of the global movement on health promotion through the contribution of International Conferences on Health Promotion.

One needs to distinguish health education from the health promotion approach. Health education strategies are usually rooted within biomedically positivist frameworks that focus on individuals, whereas health promotion strategies are usually associated with a broader empowerment agenda and consider the social, environmental, economic, and political determinants of health. However, many like Breslow (12) view them as two sides of the same coin, as the underpinning philosophies are interrelated. Health education strategies, because of their biomedically driven sociocognitive behavioral change approach, are readily accepted and incorporated into health service systems (13). However, health education can be an essential component of health promotion programs.

Another concept that combines the two is *health literacy* defined as the ability of individuals to gain access to, understand, and use information in ways that promote and maintain good health (14). By improving people's access to health information and their capacity to use it effectively, health literacy is critical to empowerment, a core element of health promotion. Health literacy thus goes beyond a narrow concept of health education and individual behavior-oriented communication, and addresses the environmental, political, and social factors that determine health. For health promotion practitioners, health literacy is conceptually attractive in its fit with contemporary health promotion, understood as a personal and communal 'asset' that can be developed through educational, organizational, and other interventions that support greater control over a range of determinants of health.

THEORETICAL FOUNDATIONS OF HEALTH PROMOTION

Health promotion program planners can easily get confused by the vast multitude of theories and models of behavior change (Table 1.1) (15–20). Strategies intended to change people's behavior can often be derived from individual-level theories, whereas those aimed at changing the environment draw on community-level theories. Theories at the interpersonal level (e.g., social cognitive theory) lie in between, exploring the reciprocal exchanges between individuals and their environments. It is important to consider various factors, such as the specific health problem being addressed, the population(s) being served, and the local contexts of program implementation when choosing a theoretical framework/model. Effective public health practice depends on using theories and strategies that are appropriate to a situation. Adequately addressing an issue may require more than one theory, and no one theory is suitable for all cases.

PROGRAM MODELS FOR HEALTH PROMOTION

Various program planning models for health promotion have been described in the literature (20, 21). Planning models, such as social marketing (22) and PRECEDE-PROCEED (23), to name just two, provide templates that public health planners can use to design health promotion programs and predict their effectiveness in a given situation. Social marketing is the application of commercial marketing approaches to the analysis, planning, execution, and evaluation of programs designed to influence voluntary behavior and involves identifying an effective 'marketing mix' (the four P's of product, price, place, and promotion) (22). Developed by Green, Kreuter, and

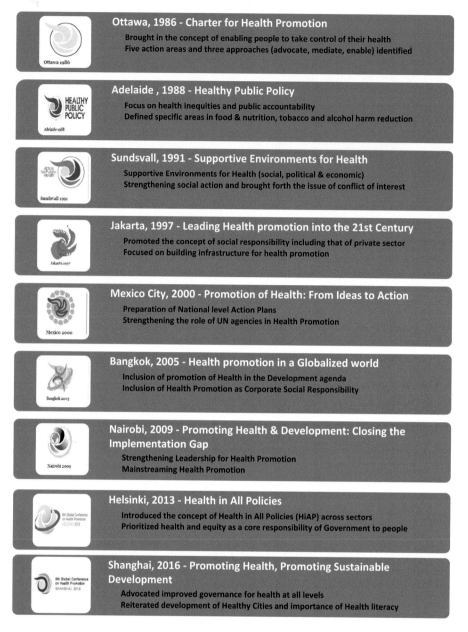

Five action areas and three approaches (advocate, mediate, enable) identified

Adelaide 1988

Focus on health inequities and public accountability

Sundsvall 1991

Promoted the concept of social responsibility including that of private sector

Mexico 2000
Mexico City, 2000 - Promotion of Health: From Ideas to Action

Bangkok 2005

Nairobi 2009

Prioritized health and equity as a core responsibility of Government to people

Advocated improved governance for health at all levels

Figure 1.1 From Ottawa 1986 to Shanghai 2016 – Conceptual progress in the Global Health Promotion Agenda (12). (Adapted from Milestones in Health Promotion, Statements from Global Conferences. WHO, 2009.)

associates, PRECEDE-PROCEED provides a road map for designing an assessment of health needs; and the design, implementation, and evaluation of health promotion programs to meet those needs (23).

PLANNING HEALTH PROMOTION ACTIVITIES

Health promotion programs differ in goals, scale, settings, contexts, and resources. Regardless of the model used, planners need to find a good fit between desired goals, available resources, and specific contexts. It is therefore recommended to use a range of planning tools, with the consensus being that a program targeting multiple action areas is likely to have better results

Table 1.1: Summary of Theoretical Frameworks and Models for Behavior Change Communication (BCC)

Level	Theory/ Model	Summary Description	Key Concepts
Individual	Health belief model	For people to adopt recommended behaviors, their perceived threat of disease (and its severity) and benefits of action must outweigh their perceived barriers to action.	Perceived susceptibility, perceived severity, perceived benefits of action, perceived barriers to action, cues to action, self-efficacy
	Stages of change (transtheoretical model)	In adopting healthy behaviors or eliminating unhealthy ones, people progress through five levels related to their readiness to change. At each stage, different intervention strategies help people progress to the next stage.	Stages in behavior change: precontemplation, contemplation, preparation, action, maintenance
	Salutogenesis	Holistic focus on health-enhancing factors (generalized resistance resources) that help one cope with and manage life and bring a sense of meaning and coherence to life.	Generalized resistance resources, sense of coherence
Interpersonal	Theory of reasoned action/planned behavior	For behaviors that are within a person's control, behavioral intentions predict actual behavior. Intentions are determined by attitude toward the behavior and beliefs regarding others people's support of the behavior. People's perceived control over the opportunities, resources, and skills needed to perform a behavior affect behavioral intentions.	Attitude toward the behavior, outcome expectations, value of outcome expectations, subjective norms and beliefs of others, desire to comply, perceived behavioral control
	Social learning/ social cognitive theory	Emphasizes the interaction between social influence and cognition, which triggers and maintains behavior change. Self-efficacy is one of the most important characteristics that determine behavioral change.	Self-efficacy, reciprocal determinism, behavioral capability, outcome expectations, observational learning
Community	Community organization model	Public health workers help communities identify health and social problems, and they plan and implement strategies to address these problems. Active community participation is essential.	Social planning, locality development, social action
	Diffusion of innovations theory	People, organizations, or societies adopt new ideas, products, or behaviors at different rates. The rate of adoption is affected by predictable factors.	Advantage, compatibility, complexity, trialability observability
	Community Readiness Model (CRM)	CRM expanded principles of personal stages of change model and diffusion of innovations theory to include new dimensions unique to communities and introduced stages within each dimension to track the progress of a community from a state of no awareness to the community taking full ownership of an issue.	CRM's six dimensions for readiness: community efforts, community knowledge, leadership, community climate, community knowledge, relevant resources
	Ecological approaches	Effective interventions must influence multiple levels and environmental subsystems like family, community, workplace, beliefs and traditions, economics, and the physical and social environments.	Multiple levels of influence: intrapersonal, interpersonal, institutional, community, public policy

than those addressing a single action area, and it is better to use strategies that favor long-term program maintenance and lasting changes in what people feel, think, and do (24). The program must be planned in a manner that provides organized and structured activities and events over time with a focus on helping individuals and those around them make informed decisions about their health.

STEPS IN PLANNING A HEALTH PROMOTION PROGRAM

An easily understandable and replicable framework for public health professionals for planning and implementation of a health promotion program uses the six steps described next (25).

Step 1: Preplanning and project management. At this stage stakeholder identification, development of a plan to manage their participation, timelines, resource analysis, determination of data collection methods, and articulating a clear decision-making process are of paramount importance.

Step 2: Situational assessment. This step involves examining the legal and political environment, the health needs of the population, and the available evidence to arrive at an overall vision for the project. Public health planners prefer the term 'situational assessment' to 'needs assessment', as it represents a shift away from focusing only on problems and difficulties to also include identifying the strengths and assets of individuals and communities that may affect the overall success of the intervention. For example, a needs assessment in an urban slum with higher tobacco and alcohol consumption, poor housing, and low levels of physical activity may bring out that the community needs better avenues for recreation, improved housing, and tobacco/alcohol cessation programs. A situational assessment would go beyond this to also identify the strengths of the community like a high level of social capital (e.g., a history of successful lobbying at the municipal level, lots of volunteerism, and one major community festival every season).

Step 3: Identify goals, populations of interest, and objectives. Situational assessment results are used to formulate realistic goals and objectives and identify populations of interest or target populations. These should be aligned with the strategic priorities of local government and the health-promoting organization. It is recommended to involve community members, participating organizations, and the workforce in the goal-setting discussions, as their buy-in is critical to the successful implementation of the plan.

Step 4: Identify strategies, activities, and resources. In this step, the results of the situational assessment are used to identify feasible strategies and activities within the available resources in terms of time, money, manpower (health workforce and lay volunteers), and infrastructure. These discussions should occur in a participatory environment including experts alongside the lived experiences of community members. A program should strive to use multiple strategies, such as combining a policy and an educational intervention. A strategy is a broad approach to facilitating change. Each strategy contains one or more activities. An activity is a specific product or service (something you do or produce). For example, one might distribute pamphlets, posters, and articles as part of an educational strategy. Tasks are part of operational work plans that assign people, resources, and deadlines to make activities happen.

Step 5: Develop indicators. This step is about choosing indicators that assess the extent to which the process and outcome objectives have been met. Indicators help to decide whether the program is effective and successful. Each objective should have one or more clearly defined indicators of success (outcome variables). Indicators can be short, medium, or long term, consistent with the objectives they measure. Simpler and well-defined objectives make it easier to develop an indicator and collect data for it. One example of an indicator could be the proportion of a population that thinks passive smoking is unhealthy. Planners also use process indicators that measure both the quantitative and qualitative aspects of program delivery. It is important to consider the source of data for such indicators and include resources for the same during the process of planning.

Step 6: Review the program plan. The purpose of this step is to review and clarify the contribution of each component of the plan to its objectives, identify gaps, ensure adequate resources, and ensure consistency with the situational assessment findings. It is recommended to use logic models when reviewing a program plan (18, 20). A logic model is a graphic depiction of the relationship between all parts of a program (i.e., goals, objectives, populations, strategies, and activities). The model should be examined to assess whether strategies effectively contribute to goals and objectives and whether the resources are adequate to implement the activities. Once reviewed and modified appropriately, the program plan is ready for rollout and implementation.

CONTEXTUALIZING HEALTH PROMOTION TO SPECIFIC BEHAVIORS, SITES, AND POPULATIONS

Translation of theoretical health promotion approaches to specific behaviors, sites, and populations poses a major challenge in the real-world scenario. A *setting for health* has been defined as

> the place or social context in which people engage in daily activities in which environmental, organisational and personal factors interact to affect health and wellbeing … where people actively use and shape the environment and thus create or solve problems relating to health … normally … having physical boundaries, a range of people with defined roles, and an organisational structure.
>
> **(26)**

Thus, a settings approach not only recognizes the context of a setting but also contends that health improvement requires investment in the social systems in which people spend their daily lives. The Healthy Cities program launched by the World Health Organization (WHO) in 1986 was the first macrolevel example of a settings-based approach (27). This was soon followed up by similar initiatives in smaller settings such as schools, workplaces, and hospitals, giving rise to the familiar terms of health-promoting schools, workplaces, and hospitals, respectively.

Schools as Settings for Health Promotion

Health-promoting schools incorporate health into all aspects of school life by integrating health into the curricula and the extracurricular environment. This could involve the provision of safe drinking water and sanitation facilities alongside school-based nutrition and screening services and skills-based health education in order to promote and sustain healthy behavior early in the lifecycle (28). Schools have also been used as a setting for tobacco use interventions. The concept can be easily extended to universities and other educational institutions (29).

BOX 1.2 HRIDAY-SHAN

HRIDAY (Health Related Information Dissemination Amongst Youth) and SHAN (Student Health Action Network) are two components of a New Delhi–based voluntary organization established in 1992 promoting health, particularly among and through youth. HRIDAY targets students in the 10- to 13-year-old age group, as health behavior is etched in early school days and can be positively influenced by providing health education in an engaging manner. The second component, SHAN, provides a forum for students (14–17 years old) to engage in peer group discussions about future health policies and programs and voice their demands to policymakers. The underlying philosophy is that appropriate information provided to students leads to increased awareness of various health issues. This needs to be complemented by appropriate skills that empower them to achieve positive behavioral change. The SHAN component imparts advocacy skills to this cohort of aware and skilled students and motivates them to become effective youth health change agents. This also fosters a sense of ownership in the program. Taken together they form a comprehensive health promotion strategy in schools. HRIDAY-SHAN interventions in the context of the onset of tobacco use among school-age students in 30 Delhi schools were evaluated and the intervention group showed a significantly lower-than-anticipated rise in school-age students experimenting with tobacco products. The intervention also reduced offers and intention of tobacco use among students of schools in the intervention group. The HRIDAY-SHAN program has been listed as a best practice model by the WHO and was recommended for global replication. It now covers 300 schools and 10 colleges in Delhi and is being extended to 12 states in India.

(Sources: 30; HRIDAY, https://hriday.org.in/)

Workplaces as Settings for Health Promotion

Worksite health programs are a combination of individual- and organizational-level interventions to influence health, and can utilize either informational approaches directed at improving knowledge, or behavioral or social approaches. Some examples of worksite health programs and services are seminars on health topics such as fitness or stress management; exercise/yoga classes; screening programs; and ergonomic design to promote health. Workplace health programs should be thought of as basic investments in human capital, similar to training, mentoring, and other employee development programs resulting in better health outcomes for employees and better business outcomes for organizations (31,32).

Life Course Approach to Health

A person's physical and mental health and well-being are influenced throughout life by the wider determinants of health. Unlike a disease-oriented approach, which focuses on interventions for a single condition often at a single life stage, a life course approach considers the critical stages, transitions, and settings where large differences can be made in promoting or restoring health and well-being. Growing evidence suggests that there are critical periods of growth and development, not just in utero and early infancy but also during childhood and adolescence when environmental exposures do more damage to health or can provide long-term health potential than they would at other times. There is also evidence of sensitive developmental stages in childhood and adolescence when social and cognitive skills, habits, coping strategies, attitudes, and values are more easily acquired than at later ages. These abilities and skills strongly influence life course trajectories with implications for health in later life. Adopting the life course approach means identifying opportunities for minimizing risk factors and enhancing protective factors through evidence-based interventions at important life stages, from the perinatal period through early childhood to adolescence, working age, preconception and the family-building years, and into older age. A life course approach helps identify chains of risk that can be broken and times of intervention that may be especially effective. The importance of adolescence in achieving optimal nutrition and its potential effects on future pregnancies, fetal and infant malnutrition, and malnutrition in adulthood is well illustrated by Darnton-Hill et al. (33).

BOX 1.3 HEALTH EDUCATION INTERVENTION

Kilkari is a mobile health (mHealth) service launched by the Government of India to help nearly 10 million new and expecting mothers make healthier choices and lead longer, healthier lives. Kilkari (a baby's gurgle in Hindi) delivers free, weekly, time-appropriate audio messages about pregnancy, childbirth, and child care via interactive voice response (IVR). Messaging begins in the second trimester of pregnancy and continues until the child is one year old. Kilkari is the largest maternal messaging program, in terms of absolute numbers, currently being implemented globally. Utilizing the penetration of mobile telephony in the hinterland and overcoming the barrier of illiteracy by recourse to audio rather than text-based messaging has helped maximize the potential to generate positive social impact through the behavioral change in the user base.

(Source: GSMA, Case Study – Kilkari: A maternal and child health service in India, 2016, https://www.gsma.com/mobilefordevelopment/wp-content/uploads/2016/10/mHealth-Kilkari-a-maternal-and-child-health-service-in-India.pdf)

Role of the Health Promotion Workforce

Developing a competent health promotion workforce is a key component of capacity building and is critical to delivering health promotion services. Those engaged in health include specialists, who provide leadership in the development and implementation of policy and practice across a range of settings; and a wider circle of practitioners drawn from different sectors such as health, education, employment, community, and the arts and sciences, and whose work incorporates a health promotion perspective. The eight domains of core competencies of a trained health promotion workforce are defined by The Galway Consensus Statement (34):

- *Catalyzing change* – developing a vision of enabling change and empowering communities.
- *Leadership* – mobilizing and managing resources and capable of providing strategic direction.

- *Assessment* – using quantitative and qualitative techniques to identify socio-environmental factors affecting health.
- *Planning* – developing goals and objectives based on the situational assessment and identifying strategies.
- *Implementation* – managing human and material resources.
- *Evaluation* – determining the reach, effectiveness, impact, and sustainability of health programs.
- *Advocacy* – with and on behalf of individuals and communities for a healthy public policy.
- *Partnerships* – collaborating across disciplines, sectors, and with all stakeholders.

Complex intervention research can be considered in terms of phases (not necessarily sequential): development or identification of an intervention, feasibility assessment of the intervention and evaluation design, evaluation of the intervention, and impactful implementation (35). These phases should answer six core questions: How does the intervention interact with its context? What is the underpinning program theory? How can diverse stakeholder perspectives be included in the research? What are the key uncertainties? How can the intervention be refined? What are the comparative resource and outcome consequences of the intervention? The answers to these questions should guide further action.

Glasgow et al. proposed a model (termed the RE-AIM model) for evaluating public health interventions that assess five dimensions: reach, efficacy, adoption, implementation, and maintenance. These dimensions occur at multiple levels (e.g., individual, clinic or organization, community) and interact to determine the public health or population-based impact of a program or policy (36). This framework continues to evolve to focus on contextual and explanatory factors related to RE-AIM outcomes, and integrate RE-AIM with other pragmatic and reporting frameworks. Current foci of RE-AIM include increasing the emphasis on cost and adaptations to programs and expanding the use of qualitative methods to understand how and why results came about (37).

CONCLUSION

Health promotion as defined in the Ottawa Charter is a comprehensive, multipronged, and integrated approach that seeks to bring about change in people's health and well-being. It addresses the complexities and interdependence of social, political, environmental, and behavioral factors impacting the health of individuals and populations. Health promotion, in the contemporary context, means creating an enabling environment through health-promoting policies and multisectoral coordination at the country, organization, village, and community levels.

REFERENCES

1. World Health Organization. *Ottawa Charter for Health Promotion*. 1986.
2. Winslow C-EA. The untilled fields of public health. *Science*. 1920. Available from: http://www.jstor.org/stable/1645011
3. Kickbusch I. The move towards a new public health. *Promot Educ*. 2007;Suppl 2:9, 40–1, 56–7. doi: 10.1177/10253823070140020301x.
4. Carroll S, Hills M. Health promotion, health education, and the public's health, in Roger Detels and others (eds), *Oxford Textbook of Global Public Health*, 6 edn, Oxford Textbook (Oxford, 2015; online edn, Oxford Academic, 1 Feb. 2015), https://doi.org/10.1093/med/9780199661756.003.0127.
5. World Health Organization. Milestones in health promotion: Statements from global conferences. 2009. Available from: www.who.int/healthpromotion
6. World Health Organization. MPOWER: Six policies to reverse the tobacco epidemic. 2008. Available from: https://www.who.int/tobacco/mpower/ mpower_report_six_policies_2008.pdf
7. Vyas M. Health promotion through Ayurveda. *Ayu*. 2015. Available from: https://www.ncbi.nlm.nih.gov/pubmed/26730130

8. Tountas Y. The historical origins of the basic concepts of health promotion and education: The role of ancient Greek philosophy and medicine. *Health Promot Int*. 2009. Available from: https://doi.org/10.1093/heapro/dap006.

9. Clark DW. Preventive medicine for the doctor in his community: An epidemiologic approach. *Am J Public Heal Nations Heal*. 1958. Available from: https://www.ncbi.nlm.nih.gov/pmc/articles/PMC1551701/

10. Glouberman S, Millar J. Evolution of the determinants of health, health policy, and health information systems in Canada. *Am J Public Health*. 2003. Available from: https://www.ncbi.nlm.nih.gov/pubmed/12604478

11. Epp J. *Achieving Health for All: A Framework for Health Promotion*. Health Promot. 1986.

12. Breslow L. A health promotion primer for the 1990s. *Health Aff (Millwood)*. 1990.

13. Whitehead D. A social cognitive model for health education/health promotion practice. *J Adv Nurs*. 2001.

14. Nutbeam D et al. *Theory in a Nutshell: A Practical Guide to Health Promotion Theories*. Sydney, AU: McGraw-Hill, 2010, 81 pp.

15. Prochaska JO, Diclemente CC. *Toward a Comprehensive Model of Change Behaviour Therapy-Treating Addictive Behaviors: Processes of Change*. Springer; 1986. Available from: https://doi.org/10.1007/978-1-4613-2191-0_1

16. Antonvsky A. The salutogenic model as a theory to guide health promotion. *Health Promot Int*. 1996. Available from: https://doi.org/10.1093/heapro/11.1.11

17. McLeroy KR et al. An ecological perspective on health promotion programs. *Health Educ Q*. 1988 Dec; 15(4): 351–77.

18. Rimer B, Glanz K. *Theory at a Glance: Application to Health Promotion and Health Behavior*. National Institutes of Health; 2005.

19. Sarver VT. Ajzen and Fishbein's "theory of reasoned action": A critical assessment. *J Theory Soc Behav*. 1983, *13*(2), 155–163. https://doi.org/10.1111/j.1468-5914.1983.tb00469.x.

20. Dubois N et al. Introduction to Health Promotion Program Planning. *Heal Commun Unit Cent Heal Promot Univ Toronto*. 2001, D:\DOCUME~1\THCUAN~1\Products\P (mentalhealthpromotion.net).

21. Shediac-Rizkallah MC, Bone LR. Planning for the sustainability of community-based health programs: Conceptual frameworks and future directions for research, practice and policy. *Health Educ Res*. 1998. Available from: https://doi.org/10.1093/her/13.1.87

22. Andreasen AR. Social marketing: Its definition and domain. *J Public Policy Mark*. 1994. Available from: http://www.jstor.org/stable/30000176

23. Green LW, Kreuter M. *Health Program Planning: An Educational and Ecological Approach*. McGraw-Hill; 2005.

24. Fry D, Zask A. Applying the Ottawa Charter to inform health promotion programme design. *Health Promot Int*. 2017 Oct 1; 32(5): 901–12.

25. Ontario Agency for Health Protection and Promotion (Public Health Ontario). *Planning Health Promotion Programs: Introductory Workbook*. 4th ed. Queen's Printer for Ontario; 2015.

26. Nutbeam D, Kickbusch I. Health promotion glossary. *Health Promot Int.* 1998 Dec 1; 13(4): 349–64.

27. Kenzer M. Healthy cities: A guide to the literature. *Public Health Rep.* 2000 Mar–Jun; 115(2–3): 279–89.

28. Langford et al. The WHO Health Promoting School framework for improving the health and well-being of students and staff. *Cochrane Database Syst Rev.* 2011. Available from: http://doi.wiley.com/10.1002/14651858.CD008958

29. University of British Columbia. Okanagan charter: An international charter for health promoting university and colleges. 2015. Available from: https://wellbeing.ubc.ca/okanagan-charter

30. Arora M, Stigler MH, Reddy K. Effectiveness of health promotion in preventing tobacco use among adolescents in India: Research evidence informs the National Tobacco Control Programme in India. *Glob Health Promot.* 2011 Mar; 18(1): 9–12.

31. World Health Organization. Second International Consultation on Healthy Workplaces (2012). Available from: https://www.who.int/occupational_health/Healthy_Workplaces_Rome_2012_Report.pdf?ua=1

32. Bertera RL. Planning and implementing health promotion in the workplace: A case study of the Du Pont company experience. *Health Educ Q.* 1990. Available from: https://doi.org/10.1177/109019819001700307

33. Darnton-Hill et al. A life course approach to diet, nutrition and the prevention of chronic diseases. *Public Health Nutr* 2004; 7:101–21.31.

34. Barry et al. The Galway Consensus Conference: International collaboration on the development of core competencies for health promotion and health education. *Glob Health Promot.* 2009 June; 16(2): 05–11.

35. Skivington K, Matthews L, Simpson S A, Craig P, Baird J, Blazeby J M et al. A new framework for developing and evaluating complex interventions: Update of medical research council guidance. *BMJ* 2021; 374: n2061. Available from: https://doi.org/10.1136/bmj.n2061

36. Glasgow RE, Vogt TM, Boles SM. Evaluating the public health impact of health promotion interventions: The RE-AIM framework. *Am J Public Health.* 1999; 89: 1322–7. Available from: https://doi.org/10.2105/AJPH.89.9.1322

37. Glasgow RE, Harden SM, Gaglio B, Rabin B, Smith ML, Porter GC, Ory MG, Estabrooks PA. RE-AIM planning and evaluation framework: Adapting to new science and practice with a 20-year review. *Front Public Health.* 2019 Mar 29; 7:64. Available from: https://doi.org/10.3389/fpubh.2019.00064

Case Study

Neeru S. Juneja

Gaurav had to leave school after his father, who was an auto driver and a drunkard, became ill. His mother worked as a maid and her income was not enough to feed the entire family.

DOI: 10.1201/b23385-4

2 Human Rights–Based Approaches to Public Health and Health Promotion

David Patterson, Sanjay Patnaik, and Nupur Prakash

CONTENTS

> It is my aspiration that health finally will be seen not as a blessing to be wished for, but as a human right to be fought for.
>
> **Kofi Annan**

INTRODUCTION

This chapter considers how international and national human rights legal frameworks can be used to advance public health. Approaches to social and economic development based on human rights law at national, regional, and global levels are referred to herein as *human rights–based approaches*. Why should public health and health promotion practitioners be concerned with human rights–based approaches to public health? First, because it is increasingly recognized that human rights–based approaches can deliver effective and sustainable solutions to public health challenges (1). Second, because human rights concepts and mechanisms provide opportunities to engage a wide range of national and international actors, including those addressing the social determinants of health outside the health sector. Third, because human rights–based approaches bring the authority and weight of international and national law to state action on public health, and can play a crucial role in strengthening accountability mechanisms.

Further, public health practitioners are increasingly expected to be aware of relevant national and international legal frameworks. For example, the Association of Schools of Public Health in the European Region (ASPHER) now recognizes competence in law, including international law, as a core competency for public health professionals. Finally, the history, momentum, and promise of human rights–based approaches to health provide a unifying vision of a more equitable world and a framework for addressing complex issues – such as intergenerational equity, the relationship between poverty and extreme wealth, and civic space – from a public health perspective.

WHAT ARE HUMAN RIGHTS?

Until the mid-20th century, international law was generally limited to governing the relations between states. The treatment of persons inside state borders was largely regarded as an internal matter, not subject to international legal scrutiny. Motivated by the devastating experience of the Holocaust and recent world wars, the United Nations (UN) included promoting 'respect for human rights and fundamental freedoms' in its founding charter, and in 1948 adopted the Universal Declaration of Human Rights (UDHR). As a resolution of the UN General Assembly, the UDHR is not legally binding on UN member states. To create legally binding obligations – and reflecting the political and ideological divisions of the Cold War period – in 1966 two separate UN human rights treaties were opened for signature and ratification. The ratification of international treaties is voluntary, however, the legal obligations they contain are binding on the states that ratify them. The International Covenant on Economic, Social and Cultural Rights (ICESCR) affirms rights such as the right to self-determination, to work, to form and join trade unions, to

DOI: 10.1201/b23385-5

social security, to an adequate standard of living (including adequate food, clothing, and housing), to education, to take part in cultural life, and to enjoy the benefits of scientific progress and its applications. Notably, the ICESCR (Article 12) also affirms the right of everyone to the 'highest attainable standard of physical and mental health.'

The International Covenant on Civil and Political Rights (ICCPR) affirms rights such as the right to life; to freedom from torture or cruel, inhuman, or degrading treatment or punishment; to freedom from medical or scientific experimentation without free consent; to freedom from slavery, forced labor, arbitrary arrest, or detention; to freedom from imprisonment merely on the grounds of inability to fulfill a contractual obligation; to freedom of movement and residence; equality before the courts; to freedom of thought, conscience, and religion, and of opinion; the right to form and join trade unions (as in the ICESCR) and to take part in the conduct of public affairs; and freedom from discrimination on grounds of race, color, sex, language, religion, political or other opinion, national or social origin, property, birth, or other status.

After the Cold War, in 1993 the UN General Assembly moved to end this dichotomy, declaring, 'All human rights are universal, indivisible and interdependent and interrelated.' Today, the ICESCR and the ICCPR each have more than 170 states parties (i.e., countries that have agreed to be legally bound by the respective treaty). Many states have also ratified other key UN human rights treaties that address torture; racial discrimination; enforced disappearances; the death penalty; and the rights of women, children, and people with disabilities. A treaty on business and human rights is under development.

Human rights treaties impose three types of obligations on states: the obligations to *respect*, *protect*, and *fulfill* human rights. States have an immediate legal obligation to *respect* human rights (e.g., by prohibiting discrimination on the grounds of race or religion in the provision of state health services). States also have an immediate legal obligation to *protect* people from abuses of their rights by third parties (e.g., by prohibiting discrimination on the grounds of gender, race, or religion by private health service providers). In addition, international law requires that states 'progressively realize' or fulfill some rights, such as the right of everyone to nutritious food and potable water, to the best of their capacity. This means that states must adopt appropriate legislative, administrative, budgetary, judicial, promotional, and other measures toward the full realization of these rights (2). This chapter focuses on the UN human rights treaty system and national constitutional mechanisms for protecting human rights. Regional human rights treaties in Africa, the Americas, and Europe reflect and extend these obligations.

In 2006 the UN Office of the High Commissioner for Human Rights issued guidance on the principles and standards states should follow in implementing their human rights treaty obligations (3). These include recognizing all persons as *rights-holders* with consequent legal entitlements and states as *duty-bearers* with consequent legal obligations. More recent approaches place local struggles for human rights in a global context. They emphasize mutually shared objectives of states and vulnerable groups in low- and middle-income countries, including in the face of private sector actions detrimental to human rights (4). Consider the legal action by 39 pharmaceutical companies to thwart the South African government's law reforms to reduce the cost of drugs for people living with AIDS. Civil society organizations joined the court action in support of the South African government. In the face of international scrutiny aided by the world's media, the pharmaceutical companies dropped their case. This benefited people living with HIV and AIDS, and eventually other illnesses, in low- and middle-income countries around the world (5).

Human rights also form the foundation of major UN policy frameworks. The UN 2030 Agenda for Sustainable Development, adopted in 2015, is grounded in the UDHR and international human rights treaties.

Monitoring and Enforcement

States are required to report periodically (typically every four years) on the steps taken to respect, protect, and fulfill the rights in the respective treaties. Each treaty has a committee of experts that reviews the reports and issues recommendations on steps states should take to meet their treaty obligations. Civil society organizations may also submit 'shadow reports' to the human rights treaty committees and thus play a central role in monitoring state compliance with human rights standards.

The general comments and recommendations of the treaty committees provide authoritative interpretations of their respective treaties. Most important, the treaty committees focus not only on the protection of rights in legal texts but also on the lived experience of vulnerable and disadvantaged populations – in other words, how the rights in the treaties are implemented in practice. The treaty committees can also accept complaints from other states, and sometimes from aggrieved individuals, about a state's action or inaction regarding the rights set out in the respective treaty. The treaty committees may issue a decision on the complaint with recommendations for a remedy. Although there are no compulsory enforcement mechanisms in the UN human rights treaties, egregious abuses may be escalated to the UN Human Rights Council (HRC), the UN General Assembly, and the UN Security Council.

The UN Human Rights Council is an intergovernmental body comprising 47 UN member states elected by the UN General Assembly. The HRC has established over 50 'special procedures' with both thematic and country mandates. An independent expert is appointed by the HRC to investigate and report on each mandate. The investigation includes country visits where possible and meetings with government and civil society actors. The independent expert reports are public documents. For example, in 2016, the HRC established a mandate on protection against violence and discrimination based on sexual orientation and gender identity. The HRC has also established a process of peer review, the Universal Periodic Review (UPR), of the human rights situations of all UN member states. The HRC reviews reports from the treaty committees, the special procedures and the UPR process, and reports to the UN General Assembly.

The reports of these processes are authoritative and public. This transparency provides opportunities for civil society engagement and advocacy with governments and other stakeholders to protect and promote human rights. Although the resolutions of the Human Rights Council and the UN General Assembly are not legally binding on states, they increase awareness of states' human rights obligations and expose shortcomings on the global stage.

As non-state actors, private sector corporations are not directly subject to international human rights law. The UN has developed the comprehensive Principles on Business and Human Rights, which identify the responsibilities of private sector actors and the obligations of states to regulate them (6).

THE RIGHT TO HEALTH

The constitution of the World Health Organization (WHO) defines *health* expansively:

> Health is a state of complete physical, mental and social well-being and not merely the absence of disease or infirmity. The enjoyment of the highest attainable standard of health is one of the fundamental rights of every human being without distinction of race, religion, political belief, economic or social condition.

The UDHR states:

> Everyone has the right to a standard of living adequate for the health and well-being of himself and of his family, including food, clothing, housing and medical care and necessary social services, and the right to security in the event of unemployment, sickness, disability, widowhood, old age or other lack of livelihood in circumstances beyond his control.
>
> **(Art. 25(1))**

As noted earlier, all human rights are indivisible: the human rights guaranteed in the ICESCR and the ICCPR are all necessary for the full realization of the right to health.

FAMINES, CHILD MALNUTRITION, AND CIVIL AND POLITICAL RIGHTS

Why are civil and political rights essential to the full realization of the right to health? Why, for example, are freedoms of association, and the right to seek, receive, and impart information as important as access to primary care? Consider the right to adequate food, which is essential for good health. Nobel Laureate Amartya Sen wrote that 'democracy is not merely a system of elections, but also one of public reasoning, which can play a robustly constructive role in bringing about changes in policies and priorities to advance substantive freedoms.' He noted that although there have been no famines in India since independence, endemic hunger remains, especially among children. Child malnutrition is a global challenge; in seven subregions, at least one in every four children under five years old is stunted. In the Indian context, Sen (7) observed:

The policy reform that is needed is largely a matter of clarity of economic and social thinking, and here public reasoning can certainly help. The Supreme Court has already identified the entitlement to a cooked midday meal as a right of Indian school children, but that right has been very partially implemented across the country [...] Public concerns can be made more effective through greater use of the opportunities that democracy offers, including quality newspapers and other media, which we are very fortunate to have. Thus, civil and pollical rights, such as freedom of opinion and expression, are as important as access to health care services in assuring the right to health for all.

Under international law, limitations on some rights are permissible to protect public health. No one has the right to shout 'Fire!' in a crowded theater without good reason. People with multiple drug-resistant tuberculosis may, in extreme circumstances, be confined for treatment. However, the human rights of these patients must be respected to the fullest possible extent. In a notable legal challenge in Kenya, the court endorsed a human rights approach and directed that the confinement of people with infectious diseases in prison (rather than a hospital) for the purposes of treatment was unconstitutional (8).

Under international law, limitations on civil and political rights to protect public health must be proportionate, no more restrictive than necessary to achieve the public health aim, and 'prescribed by law in a democratic society.' Some rights are guaranteed even during public health and other emergencies.

In 2000, the UN Committee on Economic, Social and Cultural Rights (CESCR) issued detailed guidance on the right to health (2). Other UN treaty committees have issued guidance on the right to health for different populations and health issues, including for women and girls, children, and those with HIV and AIDS.

The Right to Health in National Law

The right to health (in various formulations) is enshrined in over 100 national constitutions. The constitutions of some states automatically incorporate international treaty obligations, and hence the right to health, into national law. In other states, an act of parliament is required. These international and national legal frameworks serve to support health-related advocacy and related litigation to advance the right to health.

LITIGATION TO INCREASE ACCESS TO HEALTH SERVICES

Litigation can be a powerful tool to advance public health, including in resource-poor countries and contexts. The Indian Supreme Court has ruled that the right to life under section 21 of the Constitution is not merely the right to bare physical existence. Rather, it means the right to a full and meaningful life and includes the right to health (9).

Court victories can be empty, however, unless there are accompanying social movements to ensure the court orders are implemented. The *Laxmi Mandal* case (10) brought attention to the difficulties in implementing India's multiple maternal health programs within a fragile health system. The case was brought in 2008 after the death of Shanti Devi, a woman living in poverty belonging to a scheduled caste. She had died after being refused adequate maternal healthcare although she qualified for free services. The High Court of Delhi ruled that the government should facilitate access to health services for poor people and pregnant women. It also empowered a domestic campaign to ensure access to safe motherhood and reproductive health care services and influenced subsequent judicial decisions in India and other countries.

The decision set a national and international precedent for using constitutional protections of human rights to support maternal health rights. The Human Rights Law Network, the organization that brought the case, filed 25 additional cases addressing other aspects of maternal health in India. Similarly, in 2020 the Constitutional Court of Uganda stated that the government's failure to provide basic maternal health care services in public health facilities violated the right to health and guarantees in the Constitution of Uganda. The court ordered the government to provide sufficient funds for maternal health care services and to ensure that the relevant staff are fully trained (11).

Women, Gender, Human Rights, and Public Health

Although the UDHR proclaims (Article 1) 'all human beings are born free and equal in dignity and rights,' women's freedom, dignity, and equality have been persistently compromised by law and custom in ways that men's rights have not. For example, until the 1990s, because the human rights agenda had been concerned primarily with acts taking place in the public sphere, intimate partner violence was regarded as being beyond its scope.

The UN Convention on the Elimination of All Forms of Discrimination against Women (CEDAW) provides the basis for realizing equality between women and men through ensuring women's equal access to, and equal opportunities in, political and public life – including the right to vote and to stand for election – as well as in education, health, employment, and other areas. CEDAW and other human rights treaties recognize that substantive equality is essential to ensuring women's human rights. The UN Committee on the Elimination of Discrimination against Women (CEDAW Committee), which monitors the implementation of CEDAW, has noted that a purely formal legal or programmatic approach is insufficient in achieving women's de facto equality with men. To achieve substantive equality, states must also take positive measures to address the inequalities that women face. In other words, states must ensure both that laws do not discriminate against women and that arrangements are in place that allow women to actually experience equality (12).

CEDAW requires states to take all appropriate measures to eliminate discrimination against women in the field of health care and access to health services, including family planning. This includes ensuring appropriate services in connection with pregnancy, confinement, and the post-natal period (Article 12). In 1999 the CEDAW Committee issued a General Recommendation (an authoritative interpretation) on Article 12, further clarifying the key elements of state obligations (13). The CEDAW Committee also issued General Recommendations on female circumcision (1990), women and AIDS (1990), disabled women (1991), and violence against women (1992, updated in 2017). Many of the committee's other recommendations address the social and environmental determinants of women's health. These include the General Recommendations on the right of girls and women to education (2017) and on gender-related dimensions of disaster risk reduction in the context of climate change (2018).

Finally, although nonbinding on states, the declarations of key UN World Conferences (Vienna 1993, Cairo 1994, Beijing 1995) have successively affirmed that the right to health for women and girls includes, among other rights, the right to decision-making, control, autonomy, choice, bodily integrity, and freedom from violence and fear of violence. The power of these UN General Assembly statements lies in their normative value and the extent to which they are used to encourage and monitor state action on health. Their value must be judged by their impact on the freedom, dignity, and equality of women and girls, including in resource-poor countries and contexts. The full implementation of these norms and legal obligations at the national level requires governance structures, an informed media, an empowered civil society, and an active justice sector and judiciary. The response to HIV and AIDS provides an example of how international law, political will, and civil society engagement were mobilized to address a global health issue, including through a gender lens.

LESSONS FROM THE GLOBAL RESPONSE TO HIV AND AIDS: UNITED NATIONS INTERNATIONAL GUIDELINES ON HIV/AIDS AND HUMAN RIGHTS

The importance of respecting the rights of people living with HIV as part of an effective response to the AIDS epidemic was first acknowledged by the World Health Assembly (WHA) in 1988. The WHA urged states to avoid discrimination against 'HIV-infected people and people with AIDS' in the provision of services, employment, and travel, to ensure confidentiality in HIV testing, and to report on measures taken to protect their human rights and dignity. For more than three decades, the response to the HIV pandemic has provided the clearest and most comprehensive example of the application of the human rights–based approach to a global health challenge.

In 1996, an expert committee convened by the Joint United Nations Programme on HIV/AIDS (UNAIDS) and the United Nations Office of the High Commissioner for Human Rights (OHCHR) examined the application of international human rights law to HIV and AIDS. The resulting 12 principles, the International Guidelines on HIV/AIDS and Human Rights, describe actions for states to meet their legal obligations to respond to the HIV pandemic (14). The guidelines were referred to repeatedly in resolutions of the (then) intergovernmental UN Commission on Human Rights, and later of the UN Human Rights Council. The guidelines also provided a foundation for the 2003 General Comment by the UN Committee on the Rights of the Child, which monitors the implementation of the UN Convention on the Rights of the Child, on state obligations in the context of HIV and AIDS (15).

The guidelines have also had a significant impact beyond the UN human rights system. For example, they informed the 2001 UN General Assembly's 'Declaration of Commitment on HIV/AIDS' and subsequent UN General Assembly resolutions on HIV and AIDS. To this day, UN member states report periodically to the General Assembly on steps taken to implement the commitments made in successive General Assembly resolutions on HIV/AIDS. The monitoring framework for these reports includes the National Commitments and Policies Instrument (NCPI) (16). The NCPI also captures the views of civil society organizations on state action on key policy and process indicators.

Mental Health and Human Rights

The global burden of mental illness has risen alarmingly in recent years. It is estimated that over a billion people were affected by mental disorders or substance use problems in 2016. Major depressive disorder will likely be the leading cause of disease burden and disability by 2030. Yet, only 5% of government health budgets worldwide is allocated to mental health – and significantly less in low- and middle-income countries (LMICs). Furthermore, only about 10% of LMICs have a suicide prevention strategy even though it is the most common cause of death in the 15–29 years old age group.

There is a strong association between poor mental health and social disadvantage. Key risk factors for the onset and persistence of mental illness include poverty, childhood adversity, and violence. It is no surprise that an approach to global mental health based on isolating individual factors and delivering clinical services has proven to be ineffective in improving mental health at a population level (17). By contrast, an approach based on human rights includes a focus on the connections between mental health and the physical, psychosocial, political, and economic environment. The UN Special Rapporteur on the right of everyone to the enjoyment of the highest attainable standard of physical and mental health from 2014–2020 (UN Special Rapporteur on the right to health), noted that there can be no good mental health without human rights. He rejected the narrow framing of mental distress as a barrier to economic development and noted the strong relationship between indicators of poverty and common mental health conditions (18). A human rights–based approach to mental health invites a focus on the promotion of well-being for an entire population rather than a biomedical, disease-centric approach focused on individuals with cognitive or psychosocial disabilities (19). To improve well-being, responses need to address the social determinants of mental health and related structural inequities including poverty, gender inequality, and violence.

In 2019, the Special Rapporteur on the right to health noted the profound and lasting impact of interpersonal and collective violence on mental health, particularly the mental health of children. A public health approach to preventing violence, and thus improving mental health, focuses on addressing relevant structural, community, and close relationship factors. Structural violence stems from unequal power relationships in social structures. Violence and discrimination are inextricably linked and legitimized by societal behaviors and norms. Possible interventions include the implementation of early year and school programs, strengthening communities, changing cultural norms, reducing income inequality, and improving social welfare (19).

This approach is a welcome reminder of the indivisibility of human rights – improvements in mental health are dependent on gains in other rights and vice versa. The UN Human Rights Treaty Bodies have also referenced psychosocial and structural determinants of mental health such as participation in cultural diversity, an environment for children that is free from violence, ending violence against women, community inclusion, and eradicating xenophobia.

In 2018 the Lancet Commission on global mental health and sustainable development suggested that human rights need to be considered with respect to mental health in two ways: first, mental health as a human right in itself; and second, in relation to people living in vulnerable situations. However, the human rights–based approach goes further: it not only requires states to address the social determinants of mental health, it demands an inclusive and participatory process to realize the highest attainable standard of mental health for all.

As with other health programs, facilities, and goods and services, mental health services should be available, accessible, acceptable, and of good quality (2). The WHO's QualityRights initiative aims to promote mental health systems, services, and practices that prioritize respect for human rights, in line with the UN Convention on the Rights of Persons with Disabilities (20). India's Mental Healthcare Act (2017) was the first such legislation, globally, to reference the Convention on the Rights of Persons with Disabilities (21). The act proclaims the rights to access good quality, affordable state services; to community living rather than institutionalization; and to information, confidentiality, and nondiscrimination (Chapter V). The act creates corresponding duties for Indian states to ensure promotion and preventive programs for mental health and to allocate sufficient resources (Chapter VI). However, Indian states have been slow in meeting these obligations, which suggests that further social mobilization and possibly legal action may be required.

COVID-19, Public Health, and Human Rights

The COVID-19 pandemic has deepened crises of social, economic, and health inequities created by decades of neoliberal economic policies. Early in the pandemic, the UN Special Rapporteur on extreme poverty reiterated the need for universal social protection for workers in the informal sector, workers in nonstandard employment, and other workers without sickness benefits or other forms of social protection. He noted that unless these protections are in place, people who should be in quarantine or isolation because of COVID-19 infection will have little choice but to continue working to support themselves and their families. Also in 2020, the UN Special Rapporteur on the right to health explored how rights, power imbalances, corruption, and overemphasis on the biomedical paradigm have contributed to the spread and impact of COVID-19 (22). These reports are valuable because they provide a holistic view of the COVID-19 pandemic that anchors responsibility for the response in states' international legal obligations while emphasizing the importance of civil society participation.

Guidance can be drawn from the global response to the HIV pandemic. Consultations with the UNAIDS HIV and Human Rights Reference Group, experts from civil society, academia, public health, and other UN agencies have identified key lessons for COVID-19 from the HIV response. These include a human rights approach, centered on evidence, empowerment, and community engagement (23). In 2021 UN human rights experts appointed by the Human Rights Council called on states to facilitate faster and more equal access to COVID-19 vaccines worldwide, noting that 'no one is safe until all of us are safe.'

Climate Change, the Environment, Human Rights, and Public Health

A safe, clean, healthy, and sustainable environment is necessary for the full enjoyment of all human rights, including the rights to life, health, food, water, and development. At the same time, the exercise of human rights, including the rights to information, participation, and remedy, is vital to the protection of the environment and to address climate change. Understanding of the links between the environment and health is evolving. For example, an increased understanding of the role of adequate physical activity in maintaining good health also highlights the importance of safe places and spaces in cities and communities in which people can engage in regular physical activity. Reflecting the nexus between human rights and public health, WHO's Global Action Plan on Physical Activity 2018–2030 is overtly human rights–based.

Over 90 national constitutions recognize some form of the right to a healthy environment. About two-thirds of the constitutional rights refer to health and one-quarter refer to the right in terms of an ecologically balanced environment; alternative formulations include rights to a clean, safe, favorable, or wholesome environment (24). These sources, both international and national, provide strong normative and legal foundations to address environmental threats to public health, and to advocate for and monitor government action to ensure a safe, clean, healthy, and sustainable environment. The links between the environment, intergenerational equity, health, and human rights are becoming better understood and elucidated. The Preamble to the 2015 United Nations Framework Convention on Climate Change explicitly recognizes the relevance of human rights, gender equality, and intergenerational equity.

Challenges in the Application of Human Rights–Based Approaches to Public Health

There have been calls for greater evidence of the *cost-effectiveness* of human rights–based approaches. In 2011 the Global Fund to Fight AIDS, Tuberculosis and Malaria, a major donor for health programs in LMICs, adopted human rights as a strategic objective of its 2012–2016 strategy. Nonetheless, little funding was allocated to human rights programs over this period, in part due to questions about the cost-effectiveness of the proposed approaches. In 2017 the Global Fund launched an initiative to identify and quantify evidence of the effectiveness and cost-effectiveness of human rights programs in the HIV response (25). New measures may be needed for quantifying the impact and assessing the cost-effectiveness of reforms in laws, policies, and practices and changes in public attitudes and perceptions.

Another challenge to human rights–based approaches to public health lies in how such approaches need to be adapted from contexts where the predominant drivers of diseases (such as HIV) are stigma and exclusion to contexts where poverty, inequality, and the commercial determinants of health are the primary determinants of poor health. Greater national capacity is needed to advance human rights and other legal arguments to counter private sector efforts under trade and investment treaties to limit state sovereignty and action to protect public health, e.g., through tobacco control measures.

Finally, although global public health challenges cannot be effectively addressed without international cooperation, nationalism (including 'vaccine nationalism' in the context of COVID-19) and a retreat from multilateralism threatens public health and other development gains through the international human rights system.

CONCLUSION

There is now a web of national and international law, including human rights law, regulating state action on health. To be most effective, every national public health policy and program and international assistance initiative should be developed and implemented in the context of these national and international legal obligations. This will require partnerships between state officials, development agencies, public health practitioners, legal and human rights advocates, and affected communities.

Governments will rarely pursue sound public health policies in the face of powerful commercial interests without a broad social consensus demanding action on health. For inspiration, as noted earlier, let us recall at the beginning of this century the unstoppable combination of political will, science, law, and social mobilization that led to the stunning drop in the price of effective treatments for AIDS and eventually for many other essential drugs in South Africa and other LMICs (5). This case demonstrated that human rights–based approaches to health are most effective when supported by the widespread ratification of international human rights treaties, the endorsement of other global commitments, the recognition of health-related rights in national constitutions, an impartial judiciary and nonjudicial human rights oversight bodies, and a dynamic civil society.

REFERENCES

1. Hunt P, Yamin AE, Bustreo F. Making the case: What is the evidence of impact of applying human rights-based approaches to health? *Health Hum Rights.* 2015;17(2):1–10.

2. United Nations. United Nations Committee on Economic, Social and Cultural Rights. *General Comment 14: The Right to the Highest Attainable Standard of Health. E/C.12/2000/4.* 2000.

3. United Nations. *Frequently Asked Questions on a Human Rights-based Approach to Development Cooperation.* Office of the United Nations High Commissioner for Human Rights; 2006. Available from: https://www.ohchr.org/documents/publications/faqen.pdf.

4. London L. What is a human-rights based approach to health and does it matter? *Health Hum Rights.* 2008;10(1):65–80.

5. Heywood M. South Africa's treatment action campaign: Combining law and social mobilization to realize the right to health. *J Hum Rights Pract.* 2009;1(1):14–36.

6. United Nations. *Guiding Principles on Business and Human Rights: Implementing the United Nations "Respect, Protect and Remedy" Framework.* Office of the United Nations High Commissioner for Human Rights; 2011.

7. Sen A. Development as freedom: An Indian perspective. *Indian J Indust Relat.* 2006;42(2):157–69.

8. Maleche A, Were N. Petition 329: A legal challenge to the involuntary confinement of TB patients in Kenyan prisons. *Health Hum Rights.* 2016;18(1):103–8.

9. Dhanda A. Realising the right to health through cooperative judicial review: An analysis of the role of the Indian Supreme Court. In: Vilhena O, Baxi U, Viljoen F, editors. *Transformative Constitutionalism: Comparing the Apex Courts of Brazil, India and South Africa.* Pretoria University Law Press; 2013. p. 405–13.

10. High Court of Delhi. *Laxmi Mandal vs Deen Dayal Harinagar Hospital & Ors W.P. 8853/2008.* 2010.

11. CEHURD. *Judgement to the Constitutional Petition No 16 of 2011: Maternal Health Case Decided in the Affirmative.* 2020. Available from: https://www.cehurd.org/publications/download-info/judgement-to-the-constitutional-petition-no-16-of-2011-maternal-health-case-decided-in-the-affirmative/.

12. United Nations. *Committee on the Elimination of Discrimination Against Women.* General Recommendation No. 25: Article 4, paragraph 1, of the Convention (temporary special measures). 2004.

13. United Nations. *Committee on the Elimination of Discrimination Against Women.* General Recommendation No. 24: Article 12 of the Convention (women and health). A/54/38/Rev.1, chap. I. 1999. Available from: https://tbinternet.ohchr.org/Treaties/CEDAW/Shared%20Documents/1_Global/INT_CEDAW_GEC_4738_E.pdf.

14. United Nations. *International Guidelines on HIV/AIDS and Human Rights (2006 consolidated version). Joint United Nations Programme on HIV/AIDS (UNAIDS) and the Office of the High Commissioner for Human Rights (OHCHR). HR/PUB/06/9.* 2006.

15. United Nations. United Nations Committee on the Rights of the Child. *General Comment No. 3. HIV/AIDS and the Rights of the Child. CRC/GC/2003/1.* 2003.

16. Taylor A, Alfven T, Hougendobler D, Buse K. Nonbinding legal instruments in governance for global health: Lessons from the global AIDS reporting mechanism. *J Law Med Ethics.* 2014;42(1):72–87.

17. Purtle J, Nelson KL, Counts NZ, Yudell M. Population-based approaches to mental health: History, strategies, and evidence. *Annu Rev Public Health.* 2020;41:201–21.

18. United Nations. *Report of the Special Rapporteur on the Right of Everyone to the Enjoyment of the Highest Attainable Standard of Physical and Mental Health. A/75/163.* 2020.

19. United Nations. *Report of the Special Rapporteur on the Right of Everyone to the Enjoyment of the Highest Attainable Standard of Physical and Mental Health. A/HRC/41/34.* 2019.

20. Funk M, Bold ND. WHO's QualityRights initiative: Transforming services and promoting rights in mental health. *Health Hum Rights.* 2020;22(1):69–75.

21. Duffy RM, Kelly BD. *India's Mental Healthcare Act, 2017: Building Laws, Protecting Rights.* Singapore: Springer; 2020.

22. United Nations. *Report of the Special Rapporteur on the Right of Everyone to the Enjoyment of the Highest Attainable Standard of Physical and Mental Health. A/HRC/44/48.* 2020.

23. UNAIDS. Rights in the time of COVID-19: Lessons from HIV for an effective, community-led response. 2020. Available from: https://www.unaids.org/en/resources/documents/2020/human-rights-and-covid-19.

24. Knox JH. Environmental rights database: The proliferation of constitutional rights to environment. n.d. Available from: http://environmentalrightsdatabase.org/the-proliferation-of-constitutional-rights-to-environment/.

25. Jürgens R, Csete J, Lim H, Timberlake S, Smith M. Human rights and the global fund to fight AIDS, tuberculosis and malaria: How does a large funder of basic health services meet the challenge of rights-based programs? *Health Hum Rights.* 2017;19(2):183–95.

3 Facilitating People-Centered Health and Care through Patient and Public Involvement

Vikram Jha, Asha Kilaru, and Paula Wheeler

CONTENTS

INTRODUCTION

Globally, health systems are driving people-centered care through patient and public involvement (PPI) whereby patients, their families and carers, and the wider community are involved in health delivery, service design, and policy. This chapter explores how PPI can promote people-centered care across different health settings.

PEOPLE CENTEREDNESS

Patient centeredness defines excellence in healthcare, but a common understanding of how to operationalize it remains unclear.[1] Patient-centeredness is conceptualized in terms of patients' experience of healthcare, the doctor–patient relationship, and the healthcare system. Patient centeredness means different things to different stakeholders. For patients, it implies holistic care focusing on health promotion, and their values and preferences, and includes the patient–doctor/service relationship. For practitioners, it is an advocacy issue ensuring patients receive appropriate treatment. Patient involvement in decision-making and designing health services reflects the patient-centered cultures of health organizations. In public health, patient centeredness involves promoting health at a population level. The World Health Organization (WHO)[2] introduced the term *people-centered care* to extend this to the health of people within communities and their role in shaping health policy and health services.

Public health protects entire populations' health, addresses health disparities, and promotes healthcare equity and access. Integrated people-centered health delivery makes people and communities central to health systems rather than focusing on diseases and makes them more empowered. Moreover, health systems designed to meet the population's needs are more effective and cost-efficient, improving health literacy and public engagement with health.

People-centered care follows four principles:[3] *dignity and respect* for patients and their families; an *active partnership* between patients, healthcare providers, and communities; the *contribution* of people to the development and improvement of healthcare systems; and a *partnership* in the education of healthcare professionals. The Picker Institute (United Kingdom) suggested an eight-principle person-centered care framework for quality improvement of health systems:[4]

- Access to reliable health advice
- Effective treatment from trusted professionals
- Continuity of care and smooth transitions
- Involvement and support for families
- Information and support for self-care
- Involvement in decisions and respect for preferences
- Emotional support, empathy, and respect
- Attention to physical and environmental needs

DOI: 10.1201/b23385-6

PATIENT AND PUBLIC INVOLVEMENT

Patient involvement is key to implementing people-centered care at the individual clinical consultation level, facilitated by self-care and shared decision-making.[5] Changing societal disease patterns, with an increase in chronic conditions, led to the notion of patients as active partners in their care. Policymakers are extending these partnerships by involving the public in joint decisions regarding healthcare improvements, service priority setting, clinical guidelines development, and health services research. Consequently, government policy in places such as the UK is emphasizing the need to strengthen the 'patient voice' in all healthcare matters.

'Public', in public involvement, includes patients, caregivers, and community members using healthcare services. As 'consumers', they have choices and access to information to make that choice. As 'citizens', they have additional rights to be involved in evidence generation and service planning.

Three constructs explain public contribution to health care decisions:[6] the public's ability to provide credible knowledge to inform health decisions, the legitimacy of selected persons to speak on behalf of the public, and the power that the public wields in joint healthcare decisions. At the core of PPI lies participation at all levels of decision-making: individual, institution, systems, and policy. Participation is central to the right to the highest attainable standard of health and a necessity for overcoming inequalities. In addition, the right to health finds form in legislation and policy, and in both formalized and nonformalized structures that involve civil society and provides a conceptual basis on which PPI can be operationalized. The right to health contains four essential standards – availability, accessibility, acceptability, and quality – and encompasses resources, assistance, and progressive change to allow PPI to evolve and deepen.[7]

The evidence for PPI effectiveness is not robust, although there is a growing literature on improved quality and coverage of healthcare and outcomes. PPI worthiness may lie more in its inherent virtue in much the same way as there is intrinsic value in the right to health. Research has mainly focused on patient involvement in individual clinical decisions, such as shared decision-making. Few have studied population-level involvement, although there is some evidence that involvement drives healthcare improvement at the community level. All PPI require time and dedicated resources. Transparent and fair participation must engage a representation of stakeholders, and requires institutional mechanisms to empower participants and evaluate implementation. It must value and seek the participation of economically and socially vulnerable groups to avoid domination by the social or political elite. This includes class, race or ethnic group, age, sex, and, in India, caste. Cultural context, history, and power relations are challenges that must be negotiated. PPI therefore must be translated into procedural rights taking the form of state-driven or civil society–driven structures that include councils, committees, juries, and public hearings involving the public in planning, administration, training, service delivery, budgeting, compensation, and reform.

Ultimately, if participation needs to ensure greater democratic input from the public, then both partners need to be clear about the nature and degree of involvement and the costs involved, and plan how different PPI initiatives come together as a whole. Otherwise, there is a risk of piecemeal policies resulting in wasted time and resources.

BRIDGING THE GAP BETWEEN THEORY AND PRACTICE: IMPLEMENTING PATIENT AND PUBLIC INVOLVEMENT

Public involvement in healthcare is 'good', however, challenges limit successful participation. The following three case studies represent strong PPI implementation examples from the authors' experiences.

BOX 3.1 PUBLIC ENGAGEMENT AND INVOLVEMENT IN APPLIED HEALTH RESEARCH SETTINGS; NATIONAL INSTITUTE FOR HEALTH RESEARCH (NIHR) NORTH WEST COAST UK

In England's Collaborations for Leadership in Applied Health Research and Care (CLAHRCs) and Applied Research Collaborations (ARCs)[8] public engagement and involvement is a core principle, with a scope to involve the local communities in planning, conducting, and disseminating health research. The overriding principle was to treat residents with lived experience as equal to, albeit different from, research-based and professional knowledge.

'Public advisers', get involved throughout the research cycle, from identifying the research topic and collecting data through to coauthoring outputs. They represent a diverse community of ages, faiths, backgrounds, and languages, and have an interest in health and well-being. They bring life experiences and contrasting opinions to challenge health inequalities and translate research findings into service improvements. Individuals advise on personal experiences of service use; share knowledge about research projects with partners across local healthcare systems; and contribute to research governance, communication, and dissemination.

An internal evaluation of the impact of this approach revealed significant opportunities in research, with more than 100 advisers contributing to over 500 research activities. Researchers valued the input from public advisers, but there was scope for greater clarity on their role and better engagement and mutual trust between partners. Ensuring a fruitful partnership is challenging and what works in one setting but might not be transferable to another. However, in this program, advisers are an integral part of learning, from research to developing projects, and have led to valuable findings and improvements for service users.

BOX 3.2 PPI IN PATIENT SAFETY RESEARCH; NIHR PROGRAMME GRANT, UK

In this case, the overriding principle was to involve patients who had personal experience of hospital care and/or safety lapses in designing training and safety awareness interventions for hospitals and clinical staff. The project, underpinned by PPI, involved five streams for patient safety improvement: (1) assessing risk; (2) reporting incidents; (3) creating the Patient Reporting for Safe Environment (PRSE) tool; (4) engagement to prevent errors; and (5) training using personal stories of patient harm.[9]

A layperson panel (LPP) was established to facilitate layperson input into the design, conduct, analysis, and dissemination of all five streams.

A recruitment process using local newspaper advertisements and existing patient safety volunteer groups was followed by a selection day. Suitability was determined through an assessment of intentions, relevant skills, and experience (e.g., community or committee work), and an interest in patient safety. A range of sex, age, and sociodemographic characteristics was desired. A consensus activity was held to collate the panel members' roles and expectations to match those of the researchers.

The LPP included two members of the public per project for feedback on key decisions and issues as they arose. They recommended how to strengthen the patient's voice, reviewed results and implications for patients, and recommended how to implement findings into practice. An additional two laypeople chaired LPP meetings biannually to share progress. A member of the research team acted as mentor and panel convenor to provide training and practical support to the lay members. All LPP members were remunerated at hourly rates.

Lay members were active during the design phase, advising on the development of the safety PRSE tool, materials, and narratives for training junior doctors. At the analysis stage, lay members were involved in data analysis and synthesis.

In our evaluations of these projects, we found patients to be willing to codesign, coproduce, and participate in initiatives to prevent safety incidents, and the approaches used were feasible and acceptable.

BOX 3.3 THE KOOGU MAHILA OKKOOTA EXPERIENCE; FEDERATION OF SOLIDARITY GROUPS OF DALIT AND MUSLIM WOMEN IN THE SLUMS OF BRUHAT BENGALURU MAHANAGARA PALIKE, INDIA

The Society for People's Action for Development, a Bangalore-based NGO, initiated a process of improving accountability of health services and quality of care in seven wards of Bangalore Urban District between 2009 and 2015, supported by Oxfam India. The goal of the project was to create community leadership to assert the right to health by improving health services, civic amenities, and access to social entitlements, and to make local government accountable to community needs. Early discussions with community members revealed a widely held perception that local health centers provided poor-quality charity rather than a mandated service adhering to standards of accountability. Low demand for quality by the communities, coupled with a lack of quality improvement processes by the health centers, added to the mistrust and lack of confidence by the communities.

Women's Self-Help Groups (SHGs) in 50 locations within the seven wards were renamed 'Solidarity Groups' as they became aware of their health rights. Eventually, as maternal and child health issues became a focal area, the SHGs were called 'Maternal Health Monitoring Committees' (MHMCs) with the intent of the community to make the health centers accountable and demand-responsive. These MHMCs were localized to wards with maternity homes and referral hospitals. Interface meetings between the SHGs and the local health centers were held, supported by local NGOs. These meetings were the first experience of open dialogue with the health staff, and raised issues of service quality, corruption, lack of equipment, and the influence of gatekeepers. Eventually, all 50 SHGs formed a federation called Koogu Mahila Okkoota, to advocate for improved service quality and capability of the health centers, and with locally elected corporators to access citizen rights in other sectors. These efforts spread to include other local departments, including local government preschools (Anganwadis) to administer a food supplementation program for children and pregnant and lactating women. Through community participation, education and awareness-raising, health center meetings, establishing structured goals, follow-up processes, and reporting, these SHGs achieved great change in service delivery for their communities. Long after the withdrawal of the NGO, they remain active.

(Report – From hospitals to governance – realising health rights for urban communities – Experiences from Bangalore city, published by SPAD, spadorgblr@gmail.com)

RECOMMENDATIONS FOR ORGANIZATIONS IMPLEMENTING PATIENT AND PUBLIC INVOLVEMENT (PPI)

- Organizations should have an embedded structure, vision, and culture of PPI. Elements for a successful PPI include:[10]
  - Nonhierarchical and multidisciplinary working between professionals and patients.
  - Staff training on PPI.
  - Commitment to change.
- Appropriate recruitment, induction, and training of public participants is essential.
  - Ensure public participants represent the community and are prepared to make a meaningful contribution.
  - Develop a comprehensive engagement strategy for development and training.
  - Listen to personal views to create value for public involvement.
  - Create procedures to support participation such as a briefing pack, buddying, and mentoring.
- Make explicit the roles and expectations of public contributors.
  - Coproduce clear role descriptions for the participants including a code of conduct on expected behaviors.
- Early, meaningful, and sustained involvement is the aim.
  - Involve public contributors early to enable coproduction and decision-making;
  - Encourage continued communications with professionals and the public.
- Recognize public contribution.
  - Offer rewards, incentives, and support (e.g., travel, child care).
  - Communicate at all stages of the projects to sustain interest.

- Measure added value and impact.
  - Develop measures to evaluate the impact of public involvement.

CONCLUSION

PPI across healthcare is an important strategy for achieving people-centered care. In countries like the UK, PPI is included in all elements of healthcare, and research grant funders specifically require PPI in applications. In countries such as India, PPI is emergent with examples such as the one in Box 3.3 establishing firmer roots. Public health policy needs to expand and set standards for PPI as countries strive to achieve progress under the Sustainable Development Goals concerning health.

REFERENCES

1. Ishikawa H, Hashimoto H, Kiuchi T. The evolving concept of "patient centeredness" in patient-physician communication research. *Soc. Sci. Med.* 2013;96(0):147–153.

2. World Health Organisation. *People Centred Care in Low- and Middle-Income Countries: Meeting Report*. Geneva: World Health Organisation; 2010.

3. Nickel WK, Weinberger SE, Guze PA. Principles for patient and family partnership in care: An American College of Physicians position paper; for the patient partnership in healthcare committee of the American College of Physicians. *Ann Intern Med.* 2018;169:796–799.

4. Picker Institute. http://cgp.pickerinstitute.org/?page_id=1319)

5. Coulter A. Do patients want a choice and does it work? *BMJ.* 2010;341:c4989.

6. Martin GP. "Ordinary people only": Knowledge, representativeness, and the publics of public participation in healthcare. *Sociol Health & Illness.* January 2008;30(1):35–54.

7. Hunt P. Interpreting the international right to health in a human rights-based approach to health. *Health Hum Rights J.* 2016 Dec;18(2):109–130.

8. https://arc-nwc.nihr.ac.uk/ – accessed 22 June 2020.

9. Wright J, Lawton R, O'Hara J, et al. Improving patient safety through the involvement of patients: Development and evaluation of novel interventions to engage patients in preventing patient safety incidents and protecting them against unintended harm. *Programme Grants for Applied Research,* No. 4.15. Southampton (UK): NIHR Journals Library, 2016.

10. George M, Joshi SR. Healthcare through community participation. *Economic and Political Weekly,* 2012 March, 47(10).

4 Prevention and Management of Substance Use

Health Promotion and Behavioral Approaches

Atul Ambekar and Shalini Singh

CONTENTS

An ounce of prevention is worth a pound of cure.

Benjamin Franklin

BACKGROUND

While the consumption of psychoactive (addictive) substances is part and parcel of human existence, in the case of some substances and the case of some individuals, the pattern of consumption may cause health and social problems. A variety of products share the properties of providing pleasure and euphoria to consumers and are liable to be used repeatedly. Typically, tobacco and alcohol have an onset of use in adolescence and young adulthood. Inhalants (glues, thinners, petroleum products) are also getting increasingly popular among adolescents. The pattern of substance use varies markedly across the world and is impacted by cultural norms, ease of availability, and regulatory systems. Overall, the prevalence of drug use appears to be increasing everywhere in the world, making it a fundamental human problem. Cannabis ('bhang', 'ganja', 'charas' in India; 'marijuana' in many other countries) is the most common illicit substance used across the world. In South Asia, opioids (opium, heroin, and some pharmaceutical products) are commonly used. On the other hand, the use of stimulants (such as cocaine and amphetamines) and hallucinogens is much rarer in South Asia but is seen in other *low- and middle-income countries* (LMICs) of South East Asia (amphetamines) and South America (cocaine).[1] There is growing evidence that psychoactive substances vary markedly in terms of their propensity to result in public health harm. Importantly, the legal or illegal status of a substance is a poor indicator of its health damage potential.[2]

Substance use disorders (SUDs) are characterized by prolonged and repeated use of a psychoactive substance leading to significant impairment in health and overall functioning. The onset and progression of SUDs resemble a chronic noncommunicable disease with marked socioeconomic implications. A psychosocial approach to prevention and management is important since many family and community-based factors act as determinants of substance use, especially in adolescents and young adults. Poor academic performance, family dysfunction, and poor parenting practices have been proven to be risk factors. On the other hand, strong neighborhood support and early transition of the adolescent into their desired life course confers a protective resiliency to adolescents exposed to other risk factors.[3] In this chapter, we discuss various behavioral strategies that are known to work well in managing substance use-related issues.

PLANNING A RESPONSE TO SUBSTANCE USE: PREVENTION, TREATMENT, REHABILITATION, AND HARM REDUCTION

One way to classify strategies used to curb substance use is as primary, secondary, and tertiary preventive interventions designed for strategic time points along the progression of the problem.

DOI: 10.1201/b23385-7

Most effective primary prevention strategies utilize health promotion principles. Secondary preventive strategies additionally include pharmacological and psychosocial approaches that can delay the progression of and complications due to substance use disorder. Equally important are the tertiary preventive strategies, i.e., the harm reduction strategies and rehabilitation efforts that aim to minimize the complications due to substance use. In the following, we discuss the three kinds of interventions.

PREVENTION AND HEALTH PROMOTION STRATEGIES: AN OVERVIEW OF EFFECTIVE PROGRAMS

Due to progress in prevention science, we know what the modifiable risk factors are and which populations are most vulnerable to substance use and related complications. Primary and secondary prevention programs start early, focus on health promotion activities, and target at-risk populations. Next, we classify preventive and health promotion strategies based on the locus of intervention.

1. School- and college-based prevention programs have different types of content:[4]
   a. Training to improve communication, decision-making, and conflict resolution skills
   b. Knowledge-based training to educate and spread awareness about substance use
   c. Training to increase self-worth and assertiveness
   d. Recreational programs to foster healthy lifestyles

   Effective programs correct normative beliefs about drug use (for example, programs to correct false beliefs such as 'drug use is a rite of passage during college' or that 'drug use is common in school/college' by providing data on low drug use among peers). Programs that target environmental risk factors such as social incompetency, mistrust, and miscommunication among peers are more effective than simplistic 'say no to drugs' programs. Peer-delivered programs are the most effective. Booster sessions improve student outcomes.
2. *Family-based interventions* are interactive, role-play, and assignment-based programs aimed at promoting prosocial behaviors in the family. Interventions that are most effective teach emotional communication, consistency in the parent–child bond, and the practicing of positive interactions with the child.[5] Despite their effectiveness, family-based interventions have recruitment and retention issues due to challenges related to desirability, sensitivity to the emotional needs of families, and socioeconomic barriers to attending such programs in certain regions.
3. *Peer-led programs* are effective prevention strategies targeting youth where information is diffused by inserting it in routine conversations or in an instructive format.[6] Overall, peer-based interventions follow a heterogenous format: varied theoretical basis, different intervention domains, and a wide range of number of sessions. Reinforcement of health promotion messages has a bigger impact.
4. *Mass media campaigns and public service announcements* are perhaps the most utilized universal prevention programs. Research shows that there is limited impact of mass media campaigns, except when the context and content of messages are carefully planned, based on input from focus group discussions, and use appropriate theoretical constructs.[7]
5. *Community-based interventions* coordinate school, family, workplace, and peer-based programs, local community-based surveillance plans, and policy initiatives. For example, a combination of supportive family, positive role models at school/college, and adequate surveillance to prevent substance use by local authorities form a protective triad that can lower the incidence of substance use initiation among vulnerable adolescents in a community. Implementation requires gathering preliminary contextual data about the readiness of the community for a collaborative effort, prevalence of substance use, high-risk pockets, etc.
6. *Internet- and social media-based interventions*. High-speed internet and the growing popularity of social media offer a golden opportunity to plan prevention strategies that can be delivered in a cost-effective and convenient manner to all age groups, especially adolescents. Some social media campaigns have withstood aggressive advertising by alcohol, tobacco, and marijuana corporations. Some YouTube channels disseminate information about drug use-related harms and could be considered universal preventive techniques.

TREATMENT STRATEGIES: AN OVERVIEW OF EFFECTIVE BEHAVIORAL APPROACHES

Similar to any chronic medical illness, successful treatment of substance use disorders requires persistent, long-term efforts in the face of setbacks such as episodes of drug use following a period of abstinence (lapse) and restarting of drug use in an earlier dependent pattern after a period of abstinence (relapse). While pharmacotherapy is the mainstay of treatment for SUDs, it works best when combined with psychosocial and behavioral interventions. Behavioral approaches that have shown effectiveness include cognitive behavioral therapy, motivation enhancement therapy, contingency management program, community reinforcement approach, and group therapy.[8]

HARM REDUCTION STRATEGIES: AN OVERVIEW OF EFFECTIVE INTERVENTIONS MINIMIZING HEALTH RISKS

The key objective of harm reduction strategies is to reduce the negative health, social, and economic consequences of substance use, without necessarily reducing substance use. Harm reduction approaches often face unsubstantiated criticism for 'enabling' substance use. On the contrary, harm reduction programs reduce the overall public health burden by improving help-seeking and minimizing risky behaviors such as unsafe sexual practices, injecting drug use, and drug overdose.[9] While the harm reduction approach is mostly employed for those already using substances (often at the more severe end of the spectrum), as a philosophy, harm reduction could also be beneficial for those at the early stage of drug use. Examples of harm reduction strategies include:

- Drug substitution therapy in which a legal and safer medicine is provided under medical supervision as a substitute for illicit drugs
- Early interventions for injection site complications (such as abscesses) by trained healthcare staff for people who inject drugs (PWID)
- Providing a safe and supervised facility for the administration of illicit self-procured drugs through injection and other modes
- Safe drug use kits, containing safer drug use paraphernalia distributed by peer outreach services and made available at drop-in centers
- Overdose management services such as providing overdose education, easier access to naloxone (antidote for opioid overdose), and emergency kits
- Interventions to prevent the spread of bloodborne viruses such as HIV, and hepatitis B and C:
  - Needle syringe programs wherein sterile injecting equipment is provided to PWID
  - Information, education, and communication campaigns for PWID and their sexual partners to encourage safer sex and drug use practices
  - Organization of vaccination programs and increasing availability of screening and treatment facilities
- Harm reduction housing programs for people who use drugs (PWUD) to shelter them during periods of chronic homelessness and other social crises
- Use of random breath testing, retributive measures as well as provision of safe public transport to prevent drunk driving
- Laboratory services for testing illicit drugs for purity and contents at music festivals

DRUG POLICIES AND THEIR ROLE IN PREVENTION AND MANAGEMENT OF SUBSTANCE USE

Most countries' drug policies are as per the national objectives, which are in turn shaped by popular opinion, indigenous customs, local health and welfare concerns, and international trends and commitments of the nation. The drug policies of countries in the South and Southeast Asian region hold special significance since the region has become a hotbed of cultivation, production, and trade of illicit drugs. A 'war on drugs' stance has been the predominant approach of several countries, and it relies heavily on strict supply reduction measures and stringent penalties (from imprisonment to even the death penalty) for offenses such as consumption and trade. However, such policies have had undesirable consequences such as the expansion of organized illegal drug markets, enhanced health burden due to marginalization of people who use drugs, and increased incidence of human rights violations in the quest for achieving drug control objectives. An ideal approach would ensure a judicious balance of drug supply control along with an optimum focus on demand reduction and harm reduction measures. There is growing international consensus that drug policies should uphold human rights, make provisions for sustainable and inclusive development programs, and amend laws to ensure proportionate sentencing for drug-related offenses.[10]

CONCLUSION

The prevention and management of substance use is an intensive, continuous process. Across the three tiers of prevention, strategies rooted in the evidence base of effectiveness, cultural adaptability, and protection of human rights, including minimizing the stigma and discrimination, must be incorporated into comprehensive health programs. Behavioral approaches are an important accompaniment to pharmacological interventions. As opposed to the marginal impact of penal measures as deterrence for substance use, harm reduction strategies are attractive to PWUD and reduce the public health burden. Drug policies should aim to strike a balance between supply reduction, demand reduction, and harm reduction.

KEY MESSAGES

- The primary goals of interventions for substance use are the same as those for the treatment of other chronic illnesses: alleviate risk factors, improve overall health and functioning, and mitigate the impact.
- The locus of effective prevention strategies includes school, family, community, workplace, peer groups, and media. Balanced drug policies also play a role. The focus is mostly on health promotion principles. The use of the internet could improve accessibility for health promotion messages and treatment.
- Psychosocial therapies play an important role in reducing the risk of relapse to substance use. Motivation to cut down drug use and loss of control regarding use is targeted using behavioral approaches and existing support mechanisms.
- Harm reduction is an effective tertiary prevention approach that limits the harmful consequences of drug use and improves health service utilization by drug users.
- Governments need to formulate evidence-based laws, policies, and programs that strike a balance between demand reduction, supply reduction, and harm reduction strategies, as appropriate to their context and burden of SUDs.

REFERENCES

1. *World Drug Report 2021*. Accessed 7 February 2022. https://www.unodc.org/unodc/en/data-and-analysis/wdr2021.html
2. Nutt, David. *Drugs without the Hot Air: Making Sense of Legal and Illegal Drugs*. 2nd edition. UIT Cambridge LTD, 2020.
3. Spooner, Catherine, and Kate Hetherington. *Social Determinants of Drug Use*. National Drug and Alcohol Research Centre, University of New South Wales, 2005.
4. Griffin, Kenneth W., and Gilbert J. Botvin. 'Evidence-Based Interventions for Preventing Substance Use Disorders in Adolescents'. *Child and Adolescent Psychiatric Clinics of North America* 19, no. 3 (July 2010): 505–26. https://doi.org/10.1016/j.chc.2010.03.005.
5. Cassidy, Alyssa, and Abner Weng Cheong Poon. 'A Scoping Review of Family-Based Interventions in Drug and Alcohol Services: Implications for Social Work Practice'. *Journal of Social Work Practice in the Addictions* 19, no. 4 (2 October 2019): 345–67. https://doi.org/10.1080/1533256X.2019.1659068.
6. Georgie J., MacArthur, Harrison Sean, Caldwell Deborah M., Hickman Matthew, and Campbell Rona. 'Peer-Led Interventions to Prevent Tobacco, Alcohol and/or Drug Use

among Young People Aged 11–21 Years: A Systematic Review and Meta-Analysis'. *Addiction* 111, no. 3 (March 2016): 391–407. https://doi.org/10.1111/add.13224.

7. Allara, Elias, Marica Ferri, Alessandra Bo, Antonio Gasparrini, and Fabrizio Faggiano. 'Are Mass-Media Campaigns Effective in Preventing Drug Use? A Cochrane Systematic Review and Meta-Analysis'. *BMJ Open* 5, no. 9 (3 September 2015): e007449. https://doi.org/10.1136/bmjopen-2014-007449.

8. Blonigen, Daniel M., John W. Finney, Paula L. Wilbourne, and Rudolf H. Moos. 'Psychosocial Treatments for Substance Use Disorders'. In *A Guide to Treatments That Work*. 4th edition, 731–61. New York: Oxford University Press, 2015.

9. Ritter, Alison, and Jacqui Cameron. 'A Review of the Efficacy and Effectiveness of Harm Reduction Strategies for Alcohol, Tobacco and Illicit Drugs'. *Drug and Alcohol Review* 25, no. 6 (November 2006): 611–24. https://doi.org/10.1080/09595230600944529.

10. Jelsma, Martin. 'UNGASS 2016: Prospects for Treaty Reform and UN System-Wide Coherence on Drug Policy'. *Journal of Drug Policy Analysis* 10, no. 1 (15 March 2016). https://doi.org/10.1515/jdpa-2015-0021.

5 Social Media for Promoting Health

Gina Sharma and Syamant Sandhir

CONTENTS

> Don't use social media to impress people, use it to impact people.
>
> **Dave Willis**

- What are the various digital formats and areas one should be mindful of while engaging online to reach various target audiences? Digital allows us to create multiple formats from static banners to detailed blog posts, videos, and much more.
- Public health deals with long-term communication and outcome-oriented activities around predetermined goals. Campaigns, influencers, activities reaching patients, support groups, etc. provide opportunities and are increasingly becoming complex. It involves messages in multiple languages, formats, and platforms. In all this, there is the issue of trust that must be built.

For the first time in history, during the COVID-19 pandemic, people witnessed the upsides and downsides of digital platforms and social media. The pandemic proved to be a testing point where millions were locked in their homes, glued to various digital platforms, and constantly exposed to a multitude of reliable information, misinformation, and disinformation on public health. Social media has demonstrated to be an effective tool for knowledge translation by shortening the time from publication to dissemination and application of information.[1] The power of social media has risen during crises and natural disasters. Most communities are looking at reliable spokespersons and influencers to deliver fact-based information to the public; allay their fears; and address their concerns, grievances, and queries. It has been a daunting task for governments, policymakers, and experts to dispel misinformation and disinformation at the pace at which it is generated.

The advantage of popular social media platforms such as Facebook, LinkedIn, YouTube, and Twitter has been sharing of the latest information accessible to millions of people who have access to and visit these platforms. With the integration and tie-ups of news channels and media, people have access to the latest news as soon as it is released, unlike the earlier times when one had to watch the evening news or await the morning newspaper to access the latest information. News channels have also been using social media platforms to run surveys and polls, and analyze people's sentiments. Social media listening has become a very important tool to analyze major topics in health where conversations are ongoing whether they are about vaccines, fears around vaccination, rumors, and fears of the community. The COVID-19 pandemic has witnessed a phenomenon referred to as an "infodemic".[2] It is defined as a proliferation of both accurate and inaccurate information during an epidemic. It has given rise to the field of "infodemiology", the science of managing infodemics.[3] The COVID-19 pandemic has highlighted the importance of risk communication and community engagement, including infodemic surveillance and response, to be strengthened at national, regional, and global levels, in line with the core capacity requirements of the International Health Regulations (2005). As internet use increases, a multidisciplinary workforce, including epidemiologists, risk communication specialists, digital media experts, data scientists, psychologists, and social anthropologists, to manage infodemics will be needed.[4]

Going forward, public health processes and activities will be more in a digital-first mindset. Health promotion interventions, research, and evaluations are also rapidly adopting this medium of communication for wider dissemination of practices, results, etc. Also, stakeholder engagement and community participation are crucial pillars of health promotion that are best achieved through social media for certain digitally literate sections of the population in *low- and middle-income countries* (LMICs) as well.

The public health system worldwide has had to respond in multiple ways. The activity can be encapsulated into:

- Rapid delivery of critical information

DOI: 10.1201/b23385-8

- Tracking information and misinformation
- Care networks
  - Among health professionals
  - Connecting health professionals with patients
- Remote first public health delivery with a focus on cloud-based infrastructure
  - Health education transitions
  - Health events online

Rapid delivery of critical information to citizens, medical professionals, governments, and policymakers has been the driving focus. Even as conventional methods of digital communication were being used, there was a new development. Mobile apps for the management of COVID-19 led to discussions about contact tracing apps. Some countries did roll out the apps but the efficacy has been varied. The reasons for having a public open-source infrastructure have been discussed in this chapter and this highlights the need for such digital interventions for current and future requirements.

Equally, there has been a rapid escalation of misinformation. These have ranged from conspiracy theories to unsubstantiated cures, and social platforms algorithms have only worsened the scenario. The delivery of this has been around social networks, private chat networks, websites, and video platforms. There is a need to not only track this misinformation but also have a response back into the network. The response will need organizational social capital for the efficient delivery of the correct information.

Healthcare professionals have collaborated in unique, new ways. The rapid sharing of information, in the form of tweetstorms, blog posts, video updates, and infographics by healthcare professionals has been unique. This has probably helped providers by providing insight that would help decision-making and action. In addition, there has been a large number of trackers and research projects that were put online to maximize reach. These were developed with open-source tools and brought in a set of professionals to the medical technology space. Cloud applications were implemented, algorithms were written, and code repositories such as GitHub[5] were used in these collaborative activities.

Care networks with patients and health providers have evolved to focus on home care. It is still in its infancy, but public health infrastructure will focus on digital-first experiences. This may include information on symptoms, medicines, home processes, and emergency access to doctors via digital infrastructure.

More and more people are likely to be assisted with telehealth or digital therapeutics platforms. The care experience for patients would still need to integrate existing protocols into digital workflows. There will be devices that are likely to be available in people's homes or the immediate vicinity. These devices may be directly connected to the cloud or accessible via phones, apps, or more. This can create new ways of assisting patients. Chatbots, voice assistants, and teleconversations are additional components in the growing health and, specifically, public health infrastructure. Similarly, public health education is going to see a big transition. For now, it is online video meetings. But soon, content and course design will undergo a structural change. New skills to manage the emerging digital health infrastructure may be part of the curriculum. Augmented or mixed reality experiences will form part of the learning experience. These will be blended with new pedagogy in medical learning. A cloud-first approach to medical infrastructure means a new way to deliver healthcare learning and events too. It also means that video and audio content delivery in multiple languages in real time will need to be considered. As countries and states move to digital platforms to store the health data of citizens, privacy and security concerns must be addressed.

TOP THINGS TO KEEP IN MIND WHEN ENGAGING SOCIAL MEDIA

- *Misinformation/disinformation and fake news*. Consumers of online media should be prudent about posting and resharing information online. In 2020 the World Health Organization (WHO) highlighted the concept of "immunizing" people against misinformation during the COVID-19 pandemic. The United Nations' "Pause. Take care before you share" campaign also encouraged people to verify sources before sharing online content.

- *Growth of social influencers.* Social media in the coming years will see a growth of communities (local/national and global) on a wide variety of issues and topics. This will include a number of institutions and individual influencers. This has allowed the latest information to be widely shared by scientists, researchers, and policymakers faster than traditional channels. The growth of online communities and groups will ensure in the future that culture- and context-specific information that is relevant and credible will be available to the relevant and niche target audiences.
- *Growth of social media platforms.* There will be a growth of new platforms catering to niche audiences and various target age groups. Information will need to be customized to inform these audiences. New formats such as short videos and visual photographs are currently in vogue and newer formats are expected to be launched in the coming months.
- *Growth of artificial intelligence, virtual reality, and augmented reality.* Artificial intelligence, virtual reality, and augmented reality promise to play a major role in digital health and healthcare. Their applications and integration in social media are to be looked at in the future.
- *Storage of health and private data on social media platforms.* Privacy of an individual's health data or private information on social platforms is an issue that needs larger discussion to ensure proper laws or regulatory frameworks are in place to protect the rights of an individual or families about their personal data (identification details, health data, etc.).

Social media has a huge potential to achieve various health promotion goals. However, misuse is also possible, and users need to prevent and be cautious about it. The powerful potential of social media for health promotion should be used wisely.

BOX 5.1 CASE STUDY: PATIENTS ENGAGE

PatientsEngage (www.patientsengage.com/), an enterprise with social impact, is a patient-/caregiver-focused healthcare platform for supporting the management of chronic diseases. The platform has relevant information on over 50 conditions, over 25 communities, and over 1 lakh self-registered patients and caregivers, with over 1 lakh monthly views. Started by Aparna Mittal, the platform has effectively and successfully integrated and used social media platforms like Facebook, Twitter, and Instagram to engage, interact, and disseminate relevant health information on a variety of chronic disease conditions.

The website has been read by 17 lakh users. PatientsEngage has over 1800 articles and resources that are a mix of expert columns and interviews, and more than 500 patient and caregiver lived experiences, downloadable resources, and has started streaming webinars to reach and engage a wider population to empower them to proactively manage their health.

REFERENCES

1. Information and Disinformation: Social Media in the COVID-19 Crisis, https://www.ncbi.nlm.nih.gov/pmc/articles/PMC7300599/pdf/ACEM-9999-na.pdf
2. The COVID-19 infodemic. Geneva: World Health Organization; 2021 (https://www. who.int/health-topics/infodemic/the-covid-19-infodemic#tab=tab_1)
3. Sell TK et al. Improving understanding of and response to infodemics during public health emergencies. *Health Security*. 2021;19(1):1–2.
4. Listening to the public for the COVID-19 response: lessons learnt in managing the infodemic in the WHO South-East Asia Region, http://apps.who.int/iris/bitstream/handle/10665/345623/WER27september2021-xi-xvi-eng-fre.pdf
5. Let's build from here. The AI-Powered Developer Platform to Build, Scale, and Deliver Secure Software. https://github.com/about

SECTION II

APPLICATION OF HEALTH PROMOTION CONCEPTS AND APPROACHES

6 Public Health Nutrition Approaches to Health Promotion

Shweta Khandelwal

CONTENTS

> This is what people don't understand; obesity is a symptom of poverty. It's not a lifestyle choice where people are just eating and not exercising. It's because kids – and this is the problem with school lunch right now – are getting sugar, fat and empty calories – but no nutrition.
>
> **Tom Colicchio**

INTRODUCTION

Multiple forms of malnutrition (MOM), including undernutrition, overweight, obesity, multiple micronutrient deficiencies, and diet-related noncommunicable diseases (NCDs), coexist in many countries. Poor diets were responsible for 10.9 million deaths, or 22%, of all deaths among adults in 2017, with cardiovascular disease as the leading cause globally, followed by other NCDs such as cancers and diabetes (1). In comparison, tobacco was associated with 8.0 million deaths, and high blood pressure was linked to 10.4 million deaths. Notably, three dietary factors – low intake of whole grains, as well as fruits, and high consumption of sodium – accounted for more than 50% of diet-related deaths and 66% of disability-adjusted life-years (DALYs). The other 50% of deaths and 34% of DALYs were attributed to high consumption of red meat, processed meats, sugar-sweetened beverages (SSBs), and trans-fatty acids among other foods (1).

As defined by Mason et al. (2), "Public nutrition is concerned with improving nutrition in populations in both poor and industrialized countries, linking with community and public health nutrition and complementary disciplines." This domain spans from understanding and raising awareness of the nature, causes, and consequences of nutrition problems in society; epidemiology, including monitoring, surveillance, and evaluation; nutritional requirements and dietary guidelines for populations; public education, especially nutrition education for behavioral change; timely warning and prevention and mitigation of emergencies, including use of emergency food aid; public policies relevant to nutrition in several sectors, for example, economic development, health, agriculture, and education (2).

RELEVANCE OF HEALTH PROMOTION IN THE FOOD AND NUTRITION DOMAIN

Nutrition and policy science have advanced rapidly and provide powerful opportunities to reduce the adverse health and economic impacts of poor diets. Food choices must be strongly supported by a policy environment that enables healthy eating among families and communities. In addition, targeting economic incentives for the production, distribution, availability, and affordability of healthy food options needs to be prioritized. This reformed food system will enable healthy nutrition at schools, workplaces, and homes. A primary prerequisite for public health nutrition (PHN) promotion at the population level is adequate support and subsidies for agriculture, growth, production, storage, and distribution of healthy foods, fresh fruits, and whole grains and pulses.

Some public health approaches for healthy nutrition promotion at the population level are described next.

 DOI: 10.1201/b23385-10

FISCAL MEASURES (TAXATION AND SUBSIDIES)

The World Health Organization's (WHO) Global Action Plan for the Prevention and Control of NCDs 2013–2020 (3) proposes that

> as appropriate to national context, countries consider the use of economic tools that are justified by evidence, and may include taxes and subsidies, to improve access to healthy dietary choices and create incentives for behaviours associated with improved health outcomes and discourage the consumption of less healthy options.

The Comprehensive Implementation Plan on Maternal, Infant and Young Child Nutrition 2012 (4) also considers that "trade measures, taxes and subsidies are an important means of guaranteeing access and enabling healthy dietary choices." Furthermore, the Report of the Commission on Ending Childhood Obesity recommends to "implement an effective tax on sugar-sweetened beverages" (5).

Fiscal measures offer an opportunity to influence subconscious food choice by placing greater taxes on foods with either a high energy density and/or a low nutrient density, examples being foods high in refined sugars and saturated fats. Some innovative work has advocated interventions such as fiscal measures to try to reverse the increasing trend in obesity prevalence and other NCDs. For example, Mexico's sugar tax (6) appears to be having a positive impact on health outcomes and reductions in healthcare expenses (Box 6.1).

BOX 6.1 MEXICO'S SSB BAN AS A CASE STUDY DEMONSTRATING USE OF NUTRITION-BASED HEALTH PROMOTION STRATEGIES TO SUCCESSFULLY PROMOTE PUBLIC HEALTH AND NUTRITION

In Mexico, 73% of adults and 36% of children and adolescents (aged 2–19 years) are overweight or obese. Nearly 15% of adults are estimated to have type 2 diabetes, being the principal cause of mortality. Currently, SSBs contribute about 10% of total energy intake to the Mexican diet, more than three times the level recommended by the American Heart Association. Due to this context, public health professionals advocated for the passage of an excise SSB tax and carried out strong and focused public awareness campaigns about the sugar content in SSBs, the health consequences of high SSB consumption, and the rationale of an SSB tax (6). The government passed a nationwide one peso per liter (equivalent to a 10% increase) excise tax on SSBs. Studies conducted since the implementation of the tax indicate that SSB purchases by Mexican households declined by 7.6% on average in 2014 and 2015, even more than trends predicted.

PREVENTION OF EXPOSURE TO UNHEALTHY FOOD AND BEVERAGE ADVERTISING

There is overwhelming international consensus calling for marketing restrictions to be implemented, including the WHO Set of Recommendations on the Marketing of Foods and Non-Alcoholic Beverages to Children (7). A seminal example is Chile's Law of Food Labelling and Advertising (8). This law was implemented in 2016 with mandatory front-of-package warning labels for products that are high in certain levels of calories, sugars, sodium, and saturated fats. Also, it regulates the advertising and marketing of food products, particularly limiting advertisements targeting children and prohibiting the sale of products in schools that exceed the thresholds of critical nutrients. After implementation of the Law of Food Labelling and Advertising, household purchases of beverages high in sugar, sodium, and calories decreased by 23.7%.

PUBLIC HEALTH AND NUTRITION COMMUNICATION STRATEGIES

Health communication has emerged as an important tool for achieving public health objectives, including promoting and supporting individual and organizational change and eliminating health disparities. Recent trends show that health communication developers are turning to narrative forms of communication like entertainment education, storytelling, and testimonials to help achieve better PHN. Some types of communication methods or interventions used in PHN are as follows:

- *Nutrition education, counseling, and behavior change communication (BCC).* Although these three terms share overlapping components, it is important to understand their distinction. Nutrition education is a process of finding solutions to a child's nutritional problems together with their mother or caregiver. Unlike nutrition education, nutrition counseling is a two-way process during which the mother is actively involved in describing the child's problems and participating in analyzing the causes and identifying the available resources and solutions. Nutrition counseling is a step in BCC. Nutrition BCC is different from nutrition education in that BCC needs at least three contacts to change behavior. Unlike nutrition education, which aims at increasing awareness or knowledge, BCC is an ongoing process that requires effective communication to persuade, encourage, and support change. Sociocultural beliefs, customs, and attitudes toward food may have a significant influence on consumption and therefore the dietary status of families (9).
- *Labeling.* The WHO's Global Action Plan for Prevention and Control of NCDs (10) recommends a range of policy options for promoting healthy diets to member states. These include promoting "nutrition labelling, according to but not limited to, international standards … for all pre-packaged foods," in conjunction with a range of other policy actions such as taxes and subsidies, advertising restrictions, and nutrition education. Several international public health organizations strongly support health policies that aim to make people shift toward wholesome dietary patterns as well as encourage the use of traffic light food labeling to choose healthier products (Figure 6.1) (11). Labonte et al. (12) estimated that 11,715 deaths (95% CI 10,500–12,865) per year due to diet-related NCDs could be prevented if foods labeled with red traffic lights were avoided. This type of labeling has been proposed as part of a comprehensive policy response to the global epidemic of NCDs (13).
- *School health initiatives.* The school is often seen as an important place to intervene to help inculcate good practices about nutrition from early on (14). The idea is to provide timely support and preventive measures to improve the health of school children, which can be associated with their cognitive development, learning, and academic performance. Qualitative work in this space highlights several barriers to promoting nutrition in schools including budgetary constraints that may lead to low priority for health initiatives, unhealthy foods available outside of school, availability of unhealthy competitive foods at school, and perceptions that students will not eat healthy foods (15). Stakeholders (parents, school authorities, cafeteria personnel, students, teachers, etc.) can play significant roles in positively nudging and sustaining healthy eating habits among children. India's mid-day meal (MDM) scheme integrates the provision of a hot cooked meal along with an emphasis on school attendance (16).

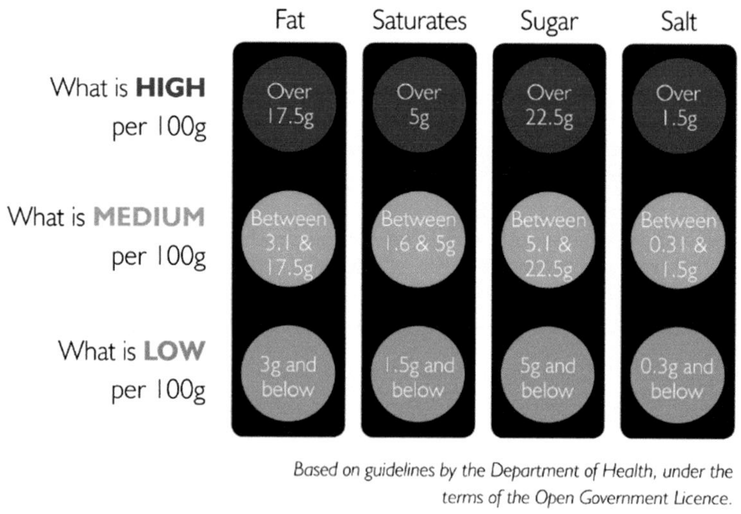

Figure 6.1 One example of traffic light labeling format.

POLICIES AND PROGRAMS TO IMPROVE FOOD ENVIRONMENT

In this section, we discuss some of the key areas in PHN policy that can be further strengthened to leverage nutritional well-being. These include breastfeeding, food fortification, and reducing fat, sugar, and salt, all via convergent action by multiple sectors for a holistic concerted policy response to malnutrition.

1. *Exclusive breastfeeding as an essential PHN program.* Six months of exclusive breastfeeding, recommended by the WHO, is regarded as a cornerstone of child survival and child health because it provides essential, irreplaceable nutrition for a child's growth and development. It serves as a child's first immunization, providing protection from respiratory infections, diarrheal disease, and other potentially life-threatening ailments. Exclusive breastfeeding has also been shown to confer protection against obesity and certain NCDs later in life (17).
2. *Food fortification.* A deficiency of micronutrients or micronutrient malnutrition, also known as hidden hunger, is a serious health risk. Fortification is the addition of key vitamins and minerals such as iron, fluoride, iodine, zinc, and vitamins A and D to staple foods such as rice, wheat, oil, milk, and salt to improve their nutritional content. Food fortification has a high benefit-to-cost ratio (1:9) (18).
3. *Intervention through a public distribution system.* Policy interventions have been shown to have an important impact on health; for example, the North Karelia project (Finland) used community and policy interventions to reduce cholesterol in the community, resulting in a large reduction in rates of cardiovascular disease (19). However, policy interventions must stimulate and support personal choices for good health, even as education enhances knowledge, alters attitudes, and helps people to acquire the skills needed for change.
4. *Eliminating trans fats.* One example is reducing or banning the use of industrially produced trans fats from our food supply chains to minimize their adverse impact on public health. Trans-fatty acids disrupt our stress, inflammation, and lipid metabolism pathways thereby predisposing us toward NCDs. Thus the WHO released a step-by-step guide referred to as the REPLACE initiative (20) to provide six strategic actions to ensure the prompt, complete, and sustained elimination of industrially produced trans fats from the food supply (see Box 6.2).

BOX 6.2 THE REPLACE ACTION PACKAGE

The WHO's REPLACE initiative provides a six-step strategic approach to eliminate industrially produced trans fats from national food supplies, with the goal of global elimination by 2023:

1. Review dietary sources of industrially produced trans fat and the landscape for required policy change.
2. Promote the replacement of industrially produced trans fat with healthier fats and oils.
3. Legislate or enact regulatory actions to eliminate industrially produced trans fat.
4. Assess and monitor trans-fat content in the food supply and changes in trans-fat consumption in the population.
5. Create awareness of the negative health impact of trans fat among policymakers, producers, suppliers, and the public.
6. Enforce compliance with policies and regulations.

Source: "REPLACE Trans-Fat: An Action Package to Eliminate Industrially Produced Trans-Fatty Acids," who.int.

LEADERSHIP, ACCOUNTABILITY, AND CAPACITY BUILDING

Evidence reinforces the importance of leadership skill promotion as an avenue to promote healthy eating and active living, which may benefit the curbing of the obesity epidemic in the short term, and the prevention of chronic diseases and mounting healthcare costs in the long term. In addition, there is also a great need to invest in capacity building and strengthening of healthcare workers especially in the area of nutrition (21). Nutritional practices don't change overnight and require sustained efforts and impactful counseling to nudge people to adopt healthier practices. The chapter author (22, 23) has previously documented the lack of capacity and attention toward PHN in India. Several stakeholders – women leaders, youth ambassadors, nutrition champions, school health monitors, wellness coordinators, frontline workers, etc. – should be nurtured and empowered further to deliver simple harmonized messages on nutrition and health across multiple platforms. Efforts to strengthen our food environments in order to make healthy foods affordable, accessible, and available to the masses should be amplified.

CONCLUSION

Any robust response to tackling public health and nutrition issues will comprise three key pillars: government action (via strong policy, laws, regulation, etc.); academia and research (via high-quality evidence generation and establishing protocols, methods, etc.); and the civil society or population at large (via empowerment of vulnerable sections, mass awareness, demanding a better food environment, etc.). The results will be suboptimal even if one pillar performs poorly or does not engage productively. PHN as well as overall social well-being are determined by a lot of factors that may be seen as outside the health system, including changing technology, socioeconomic political inequities, new patterns of consumption associated with food and communication, demographic changes, newer learning environments, family patterns, the culture and social fabric of societies, and sociopolitical and economic changes, including commercialization and trade and global environmental change. Innovative and synergistic health promotion approaches need to be imbibed that provide holistic coordinated solutions to improve PHN.

TARGETS FOR PUBLIC HEALTH NUTRITION APPROACHES TO HEALTH PROMOTION

1. Increasing per capital consumption of fresh fruits and vegetables per day to a minimum of 450–500 grams
2. Decreasing salt in all foods and beverages
3. Eliminating trans fats
4. Increasing daily consumption of nuts and seeds daily
5. Increasing consumption of whole grains, pulses, and legumes, and decreasing refined carbohydrates
6. Decreasing consumption of sugar-sweetened beverages daily
7. Increasing consumption of natural protein and fiber-rich food such as pulses, legumes, whole grains, and vegetables
8. Exclusive breastfeeding for newborns up to six months of age and continue breastfeeding up to 2 years old or beyond
9. Increase availability, accessibility, and affordability of healthy foods and beverages, especially clean water

REFERENCES

1. Afshin A, Sur PJ, Fay KA, Cornaby L, Ferrara G, Salama JS, Mullany EC, Abate KH, Abbafati C, Abebe Z, et al. Health effects of dietary risks in 195 countries, 1990–2017: A systematic analysis for the Global Burden of Disease Study 2017, *The Lancet*. 2019 May 11; 393(10184): 1958–72.

2. Mason J, Habicht J-P, Greaves J, Jonsson U, Kevany J, Martorell R, Rogers B. Public nutrition. *Am J Clin Nutr* 1996;63:399–400.

3. WHO. *Fiscal Policies for Diet and Prevention of Noncommunicable Diseases*. WHO; 2015. Contract No.: ISBN 978 92 4 151124 7.

4. *Comprehensive Implementation Plan on Maternal, Infant and Young Child Nutrition* (who.int)

5. *Report of the Commission on Ending Childhood Obesity* (who.int) https://www.who.int/publications/i/item/9789241510066?msclkid=b1e8eae0ad0311ec9bf01538660d5e0d

6. Basto-Abreu A, Barrientos-Gutierrez T, Vidana-Perez D, Colchero MA, Hernandez FM, Hernandez-Avila M, Ward ZJ, Long MW, Gortmaker SL. Cost-effectiveness of the sugar-sweetened beverage excise tax in Mexico. *Health Affairs (Project Hope).* 2019;38(11):1824–31.

7. WHO. *Set of Recommendations on the Marketing of Foods and Non-Alcoholic Beverages to Children.* WHO; 2010.

8. Taillie LS, Reyes M, Colchero MA, Popkin B, Corvalán C. An evaluation of Chile's law of food labeling and advertising on sugar-sweetened beverage purchases from 2015 to 2017: A before-and-after study. *PLoS Med.* 2020;17(2):e1003015-e.

9. Vasiloglou MF, Fletcher J, Poulia KA. Challenges and perspectives in nutritional counselling and nursing: A narrative review. *J Clin Med.* 2019;8(9): 1489.

10. WHO. *Global Action Plan for the Prevention and Control of Noncommunicable Diseases: 2013–2020.* WHO; 2013. Contract No.: ISBN 978 92 4 150623 6

11. Viola GC, Bianchi F, Croce E, Ceretti E. Are food labels effective as a means of health prevention? *J Public Health Res.* 2016;5(3):768.

12. Labonté M-E, Emrich TE, Scarborough P, Rayner M, L'Abbé MR. Traffic light labelling could prevent mortality from noncommunicable diseases in Canada: A scenario modelling study. *PLOS One.* 2019;14(12):e0226975.

13. Thow AM, Jones A, Hawkes C, Ali I, Labonté R. Nutrition labelling is a trade policy issue: Lessons from an analysis of specific trade concerns at the World Trade Organization. *Health Promotion Int.* 2017;33(4):561–71.

14. Appleby LJ, Tadesse G, Wuletawu Y, Dejene NG, Grimes JET, French MD, Teklu A, Moreda B, Negussu N, Kebede B, et al. Integrated delivery of school health interventions through the school platform: Investing for the future. *PLoS Neglected Tropical Diseases.* 2019;13(1): e0006449.

15. Lucarelli JF, Alaimo K, Mang E, Martin C, Miles R, Bailey D, Kelleher DK, Drzal NB, Liu H. Facilitators to promoting health in schools: Is school health climate the key? *J School Health.* 2014;84(2):133–40.

16. Ramachandran P. School mid-day meal programme in India: Past, present, and future. *Indian J Pediatr.* 2019 Jun;86(6):542–547. doi: 10.1007/s12098-018-02845-9. Epub 2019 Jan 12. PMID: 30637675.

17. Avula R, Oddo VM, Kadiyala S, Menon P. Scaling-up interventions to improve infant and young child feeding in India: What will it take? *Matern Child Nutr.* 2017;13(Suppl 2), e12414.

18. Olson R, Gavin-Smith B, Ferraboschi C, Kraemer K. Food fortification: The advantages, disadvantages and lessons from sight and life programs. *Nutrients.* 2021;3(4):1118. Published 2021 Mar 29. doi:10.3390/nu13041118

19. Vartiainen E. The North Karelia project: Cardiovascular disease prevention in Finland. *Glob Cardiol Sci Pract.* 2018;2018(2):13.

20. Ghebreyesus TA, Frieden TR. REPLACE: A roadmap to make the world trans fat free by 2023. *The Lancet.* 2018;391(10134):1978–80.

21. Shrimpton R, du Plessis LM, Delisle H, Blaney S, Atwood SJ, Sanders D, Margetts B, Hughes R. Public health nutrition capacity: Assuring the quality of workforce preparation for scaling up nutrition programmes. *Public Health Nutrition.* 2016;19(11):2090–100.

22. Khandelwal S, Paul T, Haddad L, Bhalla S, Gillespie S, Laxminarayan R. Postgraduate education in nutrition in south Asia: A huge mismatch between investments and needs. *BMC Med Educ*. 2014;14:3.

23. Khandelwal S, Kurpad A. Nurturing public health nutrition education in India. *Eur J Clin Nutrition*. 2014;68(5):539–40.

7 Public Health Approaches to Tobacco Control

Monika Arora, Pubudu Sumanasekara, Aastha Chugh, Pragati Hebbar, Upendra Bhojani, Mansi Chopra, and Vikrant Mohanty

CONTENTS

> Together, by working to replicate proven strategies across the world, we can save millions more lives.
>
> **Michael R. Bloomberg**

INTRODUCTION

The world has largely been affected by communicable diseases, but noncommunicable diseases (NCDs) have slowly taken over these trends with increasing prevalence, especially in times of public health emergencies such as COVID-19. Tobacco is the single most common preventable risk factor for death and disability known to mankind. Many developed countries have witnessed reductions in smoking- and tobacco-related morbidity and mortality through the implementation of effective health-promoting tobacco control policies and interventions. However, low- and middle-income countries (LMICs) are still seeing an increase in tobacco-related burdens. Control and prevention are possible by understanding trends of usage, pattern, and burden of various diseases that are an outcome of its use. This chapter focuses on elucidating public health approaches to strengthen global and national action on tobacco control following health promotion principles. This chapter outlines the burden of tobacco; history of tobacco control; health promotion approaches to tobacco control; strategies to implement interventions; and counteracting tobacco industry interference; and monitoring, surveillance, evaluation, and reporting.

BURDEN OF TOBACCO

Tobacco remains a major public health problem, globally killing more than 8 million people every year. Apart from health-related issues, tobacco has adverse social, economic, and environmental consequences at both individual and community levels. The tobacco epidemic is more significant in LMICs. Almost 80% of the world's smokers (1.1 billion) live in LMICs and the burden of smokeless tobacco (SLT) is also significant. This, in turn, worsens poverty in these countries through loss of income, loss of productivity, disease, and death.

Health, Development, and Economic Burden

Tobacco is available in myriad varieties and forms. Though cigarettes are the prominent form of tobacco product consumed in most countries, there are other smoked forms as well such as hookah, bidis (in India), kreteks (in Indonesia) or shisha, cigar, and roll-your-own cigarettes. Another form of tobacco use is SLT, which includes tobacco use by chewing (gutkha, khaini, etc.)

DOI: 10.1201/b23385-11

or snuff and tooth powder. SLT is produced and used in Southeast Asia but is currently reported to be used in 127 countries (1). LMICs such as India report SLT to be the most prominent form of tobacco use contributing to 77,000 new oral cancer cases annually with 70% of cases reported in the advanced stages (2). Tobacco use is an established major risk factor causing NCDs, which is a leading cause of death, globally. It is estimated that 12% of all deaths are attributable to tobacco use globally.

Health Effects of Tobacco

Of more than 7000 chemicals in tobacco smoke, at least 250 are known to be harmful, and 70 are known to be carcinogenic (3). Tobacco smoke released by smokers contains nicotine and other toxic chemicals, which adversely impact the health of nonsmoking bystanders or spouses, thus, requiring health promotion interventions. Smoking can be an individual choice, but harming others' health due to one's smoking habit is a human rights issue and requires tackling tobacco control as a public health issue.

According to the International Agency for Research on Cancer (IARC) monograph, there is sufficient evidence that tobacco causes cancer of the lung; oral cavity; naso-, oro-, and hypopharynx, nasal cavity, and paranasal sinuses; larynx; esophagus; stomach; pancreas; liver; kidney (body and pelvis); ureter; urinary bladder; uterine cervix; and bone marrow (myeloid leukemia).

Apart from cancers, tobacco is the chief cause of long-term adverse effects including precancerous conditions, cardiovascular disease, chronic obstructive pulmonary disease (COPD), eye diseases, rheumatoid arthritis, bone health (low bone density), and reproductive health effects.

Tobacco disproportionally impacts the poor, as consumption is higher among those of lower socioeconomic status and less educated, thus, hampering development.

HISTORY OF TOBACCO CONTROL

The first report by the Surgeon General on smoking and health marked a turning point in the history of tobacco control. The report was issued by U.S. Surgeon General Luther L. Terry in 1964 who appointed an expert committee to submit a report to review and evaluate the current data on smoking and health. The report was published under the title "Smoking and Health: Report of the Advisory Committee to the Surgeon General of the United States." This was the first of a series of reports on smoking and health issued by the U.S. Surgeon General's office. This landmark report concluded that cigarette smoking is a health hazard and a cause of lung cancer in men and a suspected cause for the same in women.

The next milestone in tobacco control was the establishment of the World Health Organization's Framework Convention on Tobacco Control (WHO FCTC). The convention was a response to the globalization of the tobacco epidemic and reaffirms the right of all people to the highest standards of health. The FCTC negotiation process required considerable advocacy from multiple stakeholders and multisectoral convergence following principles and strategies of health promotion that successfully led to the finalization of the treaty draft. The FCTC is now a tool for promoting health through proper implementation and monitoring. The WHO FCTC was adopted by the World Health Assembly on 21 May 2003 and entered into force on 27 February 2005. Currently, there are 182 parties of the WHO FCTC covering over 90% of the world's population.

In contemporary times, when nicotine products are being introduced, reducing tobacco and nicotine use requires two-pronged action: promoting cessation among current tobacco users, and preventing new nicotine and novel electronic nicotine products from entering the market (according to their context) by banning them. For example, the countries of India, Brazil, and Thailand have successfully introduced policies that prohibit the manufacture, sale, and storage of e-cigarettes and other electronic nicotine delivery devices.

This two-pronged strategy requires health promotion interventions targeting three levels: individual, community, and larger policy environment. Reaching individuals by motivational interviewing and promoting cessation, while public education through warnings on tobacco packages and mass media interventions will change social norms and denormalize tobacco use. To bring this change at the individual and community level, it is crucial to have conducive tobacco control policies: raising taxes on tobacco products, protecting nonusers from exposure to secondhand smoke and the passive impact of SLT use, and advertising bans. Advertising bans necessitate multisectoral coordination as implementation requires action from the non-health sector (e.g., finance, information, and broadcasting).

The WHO FCTC acts as a foundation for countries to implement and manage tobacco control through Articles 6–14 for core demand reduction provisions, Articles 15–17 for core supply reduction provisions, and Articles 20–22 for addressing the exchange of information as well as scientific and technical cooperation. The WHO introduced MPOWER measures to correspond with one or more of the WHO FCTC articles to assist in demand reduction of tobacco at a country level. MPOWER stands for: **m**onitor tobacco use and prevention policies; **p**rotect people from tobacco smoke; **o**ffer help to quit tobacco use; **w**arn about the dangers of tobacco; **e**nforce bans on tobacco advertising, promotion, and sponsorship; and **r**aise taxes on tobacco.

BOX 7.1 ADVOCACY FOR SUCCESSFUL TOBACCO CONTROL: CASE STUDY FROM SRI LANKA

Tobacco control became a focus officially in Sri Lanka with the establishment of the Presidential Task Force on Alcohol and Tobacco in 1995. The Alcohol and Drug Information Centre (ADIC), the leading civil society organization working for tobacco and alcohol control, began discussions with the public and politicians in 1990 on the importance of a tobacco and alcohol control policy, conducted workshops for nongovernmental organizations and community-based organizations and organized public campaigns to create a demand, and advocated with politicians for such a policy. After establishing the Presidential Task Force in 1995, a model policy was developed with the contribution of multidisciplinary experts and was handed over to the Presidential Task Force by civil society groups. In 1997, the Presidential Task Force handed over a draft policy to the president. Even though the bill was presented to the cabinet in 2000, up to 2005 there was no progress due to industry interference. In 2005, the bill reemerged as a private member bill, leading to the Minister of Health presenting the bill through its ministry. This bill was challenged in the Supreme Court of Sri Lanka by the industry. After winning the case the bill was presented to the parliament by the Minister of Health, and the National Authority on Tobacco and Alcohol Act (No. 27 of 2006) came into power. The policy was a result of 16 years of continued effort from civil society activists, academics, and professionals of the country.

Tobacco is a product with no true revenue, as the cost is always greater than any revenue from taxes. Therefore, the benefits of tobacco control are immense for the health and economy of a country. Preventing premature deaths caused by tobacco through NCDs itself saves the workforce of a country and maximizes productivity. Effective tobacco control also protects the environment from the harms of tobacco cultivation and pollution from tobacco smoke and cigarette butts. Finally, as any form of addiction including smoking results in loss of freedom and happiness, effective tobacco control increases the quality of life of the whole population.

TOBACCO CONTROL INTERVENTIONS: HEALTH PROMOTION APPROACHES

Comprehensive health promotion programs aim to deformalize tobacco use behavior in the community and, therefore, are an effective preventive measure for overall tobacco control. These health promotion activities can be aimed at tobacco control by multilevel interventions at three levels: individual, community, and policy, using MPOWER strategies such as tobacco taxation; school health programs; pictorial health warnings (PHWs); bans on tobacco advertisement, promotion, and sponsorship; and restricting tobacco access to minors. The framework is provided in Annexure 1.

M: Monitor Tobacco Use and Prevention Policies

Robust surveillance and monitoring systems help understand the trends and patterns of tobacco usage, enforcement of tobacco control measures, expenditure on tobacco products, likelihood of initiation, quitting, and other aspects related to tobacco use. These data are useful for researchers, program managers, and implementers at the national level to identify areas of improvement and strengthen program implementation. At the global level, the WHO's Tobacco Free Initiative and the US Centers for Disease Control together launched the Global Tobacco Surveillance System (GTSS). The GTSS is the largest public health surveillance system with its surveys being administered in over 185 countries. The GTSS consists of the Global Youth Tobacco Survey (GYTS), Global Adult Tobacco Survey (GATS), Global School Personnel Survey (GSPS), Global Health Professional Student Survey (GHPSS), and the Tobacco Questions for Surveys (TQS). The interactive web portal of GTSS provides the most comprehensive, reliable, and comparable global data related to tobacco control. Several countries have completed two or more cycles of these large-scale representative surveys providing rich data to assess temporal patterns. The portal also provides reports, fact sheets, and data sets for the aforementioned various surveys. Some global and national platforms for the exchange of information include the World Conference on Tobacco or Health (WCTOH) and the National Conference on Tobacco or Health (NCTOH).

School-based health programs are one of the most effective ways to comprehend and monitor tobacco use at a community level. Schools are an ideal setting to implement health programs and prevent uptake among adolescents and youth. An Indian study conducted by Arora et al. reported that peer-led interventions alongside multicomponent, health promotion theory-based interventions reduced tobacco prevalence in two cities in India (4).

Looking at prevention policies, health promotion interventions to reduce the supply of tobacco products have also shown effectiveness in reducing tobacco consumption. For example, a ban on the sale of tobacco products to minors (below the age of 18 years) is one such measure and has reduced tobacco initiation among young adults in many countries. Other ways are to eliminate the illicit trade of tobacco products, crop substitution, and elimination of government subsidies for tobacco farming.

P: Protect People from Tobacco Smoke

As per the WHO's Global Health Observatory, secondhand smoke causes an estimated 600,000 premature deaths worldwide (64% women and 40% children). Consequently, comprehensive smoke-free policies at the national level that prohibit smoking in public places (including the home, school, workplace, or public places) have been effective to protect nonusers from secondhand smoke exposure. Smoke-free policies have also been shown to reduce the social acceptability of smoking, reduce smoking initiation among young adults, and increase smokers' efforts to quit smoking.

At the community level, no tobacco use norms in families and communities play a significant role in supporting healthy habits among adolescents and youths. A community-based tobacco cessation approach has also been found to be beneficial in India, showing a significant reduction in tobacco use among adolescents in the intervention group as compared to the control group (5).

Capacity building can be essential for effective tobacco control and is a wise investment for every country to meet this approach of the MPOWER strategy. Engaging individuals, as well as civil society organizations and building their capacities for effective tobacco control, can support national-level initiatives and programs.

O: Offer Help to Quit Tobacco Use

Offering help to tobacco users by providing cessation services is vital for tobacco control. Tobacco control interventions are of two types: nonpharmacological and pharmacological. At the national level, cessation services like national toll-free quit lines and mCessation are available to aid in quitting the use of tobacco. Additionally, tobacco cessation support can be provided at primary healthcare facilities at the community level, along with the provision of cessation clinics. At the individual level, behavioral change interventions (such as the transtheoretical model, health belief model, and/or social cognitive/learning theory) and nonpharmacological interventions focus on changing the behavior toward tobacco use by motivation, self-efficacy, consideration of barriers and benefits to change, subjective norms, attitudes, and cues to actions through cognitive behavioral therapy, self-help manuals, and counseling (brief advice to quit). Pharmacological interventions are provided to tobacco users by trained healthcare professionals such as nicotine replacement therapy (NRT), which is the most widely prescribed treatment to help tobacco users quit. Studies have shown that the chances of quitting tobacco increase by 50%–70% when using NRT (6). Other pharmacological drugs include bupropion, varenicline, nortriptyline, and clonidine.

BOX 7.2 STRENGTHENING CAPACITY BUILDING ON TOBACCO CESSATION RESEARCH, TRAINING, AND PRACTICE IN INDIA AND INDONESIA

Project Quit Tobacco International (QTI) was implemented in India (two states: Kerala and Karnataka) and Indonesia (four medical colleges) following an integrated approach to build capacity for tobacco cessation. Three areas covered in Project QTI were tobacco cessation training in medical colleges, the smoke-free home initiative, and smoking cessation among diabetes patients. A total of 15 modules, including a training component on tobacco cessation for the undergraduate medical curriculum in India, were developed and implemented. QTI was successful in incorporating tobacco education in the undergraduate medical curriculum of two health universities in Kerala and Karnataka, India. As a part of the community outreach smoke-free home initiative, a survey was conducted to assess the prevalence of secondhand smoke exposure at the household level, following which the intervention was implemented through Kudumbasree, a large women's organization in Kerala, and in Indonesia. The change in prevalence of smokers not smoking inside their homes increased from 11% to 54% post-intervention. Another component of the project focused on conducting a randomized controlled trial to compare the effectiveness of a strong diabetes-specific cessation message delivery by doctors and diabetes-specific cessation counseling by a non-doctor health professional on tobacco quit rates. Favorable results for quitting and cessation were observed.

W: Warn About Dangers of Tobacco

Health warning labels on tobacco products constitute the most cost-effective tool for educating tobacco users (both smokers and SLT users) and nonsmokers about the health risks of tobacco use and increase the attempts to quit. Consequently, WHO FCTC recommends member states implement large, rotating health warnings on all tobacco product packages (Article 11 of FCTC). Thus, tobacco packages in most countries carry health warnings; however, the position, size, and general strength of these warnings vary considerably across jurisdictions. Having large PHWs with plain tobacco packaging, also known as generic, neutral standardized, or homogeneous packaging, is effective in reducing the appeal of tobacco products and increasing the noticeability of PHWs.

BOX 7.3 AUSTRALIA'S EXPERIENCE WITH PLAIN PACKAGING OF TOBACCO PRODUCTS

Australia was the first country in the world to introduce plain packaging on tobacco products, with all packets being sold in logo-free, drab, dark brown packaging since December 1, 2012. As a result of plain packaging, smokers in Australia noticed PHWs on the packs, which motivated them to quit tobacco. Plain packaging also made Australians dislike the products and, therefore, reduced the appeal of tobacco products among both tobacco users and nonusers.

At the community level, mass media campaigns (through television, radio, newspapers posters, booklets, etc.) on tobacco control provide an opportunity to spread well-defined, focused messages to raise awareness about tobacco use to a large population. The literature shows that comprehensive tobacco control programs, which include mass media campaigns, can be effective in changing tobacco use behavior among adults.

E: Enforce Bans on Tobacco Advertising, Promotion, and Sponsorship

BOX 7.4 STRINGENT TOBACCO-FREE FILM AND TV RULES IN INDIA

India is one of the earliest signatories to the WHO FCTC and has strengthened tobacco control efforts in the country, including laws prohibiting tobacco advertising, promotions, and sponsorships. In 2003, the Cigarette and Other Tobacco Products (Prohibition of Advertisement and Regulation of Trade and Commerce, Production, Supply and

Distribution) Act (COTPA Act) was passed to enforce tobacco control legislation. Section 5 of COTPA bans tobacco promotion, direct and indirect advertising of tobacco products, and event sponsorship by tobacco marketers. However, research showed that after the introduction of COTPA, the placement of tobacco products in Indian films, particularly Bollywood films, increased. Therefore, due to increased exposure to tobacco in films, a blanket ban on the depiction of smoking scenes and use of other tobacco products in films and television programs was introduced in India in 2005. Subsequently, in 2011 and 2012, the Government of India introduced stringent tobacco-free film rules to regulate the depiction of tobacco imagery in all films screened across India, which has been evaluated to show a reduction in tobacco use exposure through films and TV programs (7).

A ban on tobacco advertising, promotion, and sponsorship (TAPS) is one of the effective ways to reduce tobacco consumption. High-income countries (HICs) that have already introduced a TAPS ban show an average of 7% reduction in tobacco consumption (8). Research shows that about one-third of youth initiate tobacco use as a result of exposure to TAPS (9). One of the most evident forms of TAPS is through media (e.g., in films, television programs, and series shown on on-demand streaming platforms). Tobacco advertising, through various media, creates positive product imagery or associations in the minds of young people. New media alongside streaming platforms are now flouting TAPS bans around the world and undoing all positive impacts achieved so far from implementing Article 12 of the FCTC.

R: Raise Taxes on Tobacco

Raising the price of tobacco and its products, mainly through tax increases, is one of the most cost-effective measures to reduce consumption. Tobacco use leads to considerable economic loss, in the form of healthcare expenditure to treat diseases caused by active or passive tobacco use. Therefore, a variety of taxes (such as excise duty, customs duty, value-added tax, general sales or consumption tax, and other country-specific taxes) can be applied to tobacco and its various products. This results in reducing the affordability of tobacco products for its consumers and thereby reducing demand. Studies have shown that a 10% increase in the prices of tobacco products can reduce tobacco use by 5% and 4% on average in LMICs and HICs, respectively (10). Moreover, young people, minorities, and low-income tobacco users are more likely to quit, reduce tobacco consumption, and prevent youth from tobacco initiation in response to price increases. This leads to significant health benefits and a reduction in health inequalities.

One such example to showcase the effectiveness of the increase in taxes on tobacco products has been seen in the United Kingdom, wherein the young and poor were most likely to use cheap tobacco products, which were likely to drive inequalities in smoking in the country. Therefore, in May 2017, a minimum excise tax on tobacco was introduced via the finance bill in the United Kingdom. This successfully demonstrated that increasing tobacco taxes did not lead to illicit trade contrary to tobacco industry claims.

STRATEGIES TO IMPLEMENT INTERVENTIONS

Building institutional capacity within a country is essential for the long-term sustainability of tobacco control interventions. Following are a few strategies through which the aforementioned interventions can be successfully implemented.

1. *Developing an action plan for tobacco control based on the multisectoral convergence model.* The Ministry of Health must spearhead the process of developing the capacity for undertaking tobacco control measures. A successful national plan of action to control the tobacco epidemic also requires multistakeholder efforts beyond the health sector. The experience of many countries with progressive tobacco control programs indicates that it is best to establish a multisectoral national committee or task force at various administrative levels (at a national, subnational, or district level) in order to set up an appropriate plan for undertaking comprehensive tobacco control measures. A national multisectoral action plan for NCD prevention and control exists in many countries and tackles tobacco as an NCD risk factor and enlists activities to be implemented for achieving the target of a 30% relative reduction in the prevalence of tobacco use by 2025.

2. *Establishing an effective infrastructure for tobacco control programs.* As the development of a national plan of action unfolds, it is important to establish an effective infrastructure for implementing tobacco control programs. The established infrastructure should have sufficient human resources, budget, and other basic resources (office space, stationery, etc.).
3. *Forming effective partnerships: Adopting a whole-of-community approach.* As the development of a national plan of action unfolds, it is important to establish an effective infrastructure for implementing tobacco control programs. The established infrastructure should have sufficient human resources, budget, and other basic resources (office space, stationery, etc.). Partnerships with the health sector (with different stakeholders such as the Ministry of Health, civil society representatives, academicians) and beyond the health sector, including the Ministry of Finance, Ministry of Education, and other ministries, are vital for effective tobacco control.
4. *Training and education.* Successful implementation of tobacco control measures largely depends on the availability and quality of human resources. Capacity building is essential for effective tobacco control and is a wise investment for every country. Engaging civil society organizations and other stakeholders and building their capacities for effective tobacco control can support national-level initiatives and programs.
5. *Communication and public awareness to build critical mass.* It is critical to counteract the marketing strategies of the tobacco industry by devising a strategic communication and public awareness plan to build a mass of public supporters for tobacco control. Growing evidence also suggests social marketing is a powerful tool for achieving behavior change and, thus, can be strategically utilized for implementing tobacco control interventions.
6. *Legislative and regulatory measures.* A comprehensive tobacco control legislation aligned with the articles of the FCTC offers effective health promotion interventions for implementing tobacco control policies.

COUNTERING THE TOBACCO INDUSTRY

The tobacco industry is unique, as its products are lethal to consumers when consumed as prescribed by the manufacturers. The industry is also unique in its behavior. There is extensive documentation on how the tobacco industry has for a long time employed several tactics for influencing public health policies related to tobacco in ways that undermine the intent and implementation of these policies. This is what is referred to as the tobacco industry interference. The industry's tactics include but are not limited to intelligence gathering, public relations, political funding, lobbying, consultancy, funding science/research, use of seemingly independent third parties, intimidation, litigation, philanthropy, smuggling, and corporate social responsibilities (11).

Hence, preventing and countering tobacco industry interference in the tobacco control policy is crucial for effective tobacco control. Article 5.3 of the FCTC specifically prescribes that "in setting and implementing their public health policies with respect to tobacco control, Parties shall act to protect these policies from commercial and other vested interests of the tobacco industry in accordance with national law." It offers guidance and tools to governments in preventing tobacco industry interference. Implementation of Article 5.3 has been shown to help counter tobacco industry interference. However, globally, the implementation of Article 5.3 remains suboptimal (12).

Monitoring the tobacco industry (tactics, interference) is crucial to identify and counter industry interference in tobacco control, with many initiatives implemented across several countries, at national, regional, and global levels to monitor tobacco industry tactics and interference. Furthermore, civil society organizations have played a crucial role in monitoring and countering tobacco industry interference, such as periodic assessment of Article 5.3 implementation in countries of the Association of Southeast Asian Nations (ASEAN) through the use of a tobacco industry interference index, advocacy with government agencies, (public interest) litigations, use of media, and social mobilization.

MONITORING, SURVEILLANCE, EVALUATION, AND REPORTING

Robust surveillance and monitoring systems help understand the trends and patterns of tobacco usage, enforcement of tobacco control measures, expenditure on tobacco products, likelihood of initiation, quitting, and other aspects related to tobacco use. These data are useful for researchers, program managers, and implementers to identify areas of improvement and strengthen program implementation. As stated earlier, national-level surveillance systems/surveys provide rich data to assess tobacco use patterns and trends. In addition, conferences conducted on global and national platforms allow relevant stakeholders to come together to exchange evidence-based information for tobacco control.

CONCLUSION

Research, surveillance, implementation of evidence-based interventions, and evaluation of tobacco control programs in developed countries have successfully lowered the tobacco burden in the global north, however, interventions in LMICs still need to follow effective designing, implementation, and evaluation of tobacco control programs and policies following health promotion principles and strategies. This will go a long way in protecting LMIC populations from the dangers of the tobacco epidemic.

REFERENCES

1. Siddiqi K, Husain S, Vidyasagaran A, Readshaw A, Mishu M, Sheikh A. Global burden of disease due to smokeless tobacco consumption in adults: An updated analysis of data from 127 countries. *BMC Med.* 2020;18(1): 1–22.

2. Borse V, Konwar A, Buragohain P. Oral cancer diagnosis and perspectives in India. *Sensors Int.* 2020;1:100046.

3. National Cancer Institute (NCI). Harms of Cigarette Smoking and Health Benefits of Quitting. 2007, Available from: https://www.cancer.gov/about-cancer/causes-prevention/risk/tobacco/cessation-fact-sheet#what-harmful-chemicals-does-tobacco-smoke-contain

4. Arora M, Stigler MH, Reddy KS. Effectiveness of health promotion in preventing tobacco use among adolescents in India: Research evidence informs the National Tobacco Control Programme in India. *Global Health Promotion.* 2011;18(1):9–12.

5. Arora M, Mathur MR, Singh N. A framework to prevent and control tobacco among adolescents and children: Introducing the IMPACT Model. *India J Pediatr.* 2012;80(1) Supplement 1:S55–S62.

6. Silagy C, Mant D, Fowler G, Lancaster T. Nicotine replacement therapy for smoking cessation. *Cochrane Database Syst Rev.* 2000;(2):CD000146.

7. Nazar GP, Arora M, Sharma N, Shrivastava S, Rawal T, Chugh A, Sinha P, Munish VG, Tullu FT, Schotte K, Polansky JR. Changes in tobacco depictions after implementation of tobacco-free film and TV rules in Bollywood films in India: A trend analysis. *Tobacco Control.* 2021 Jul 26. https://doi.org/10.1136/tobaccocontrol-2021-056629

8. World Health Organization. Tobacco Free Initiative: Enforce bans on tobacco advertising, promotion and sponsorship [Internet]. Available from: https://www.who.int/tobacco/mpower/enforce/en/index3.html

9. DiFranza JR, Wellman RJ, Sargent JD, Weitzman M, Hipple BJ, Winickoff JP. Tobacco promotion and the initiation of tobacco use: Assessing the evidence for causality. *Pediatrics.* 2006;117(6):e1237–e1248.

10. Chaloupka FJ, Yurekli A, Fong GT. Tobacco taxes as a tobacco control strategy. *Tob Control.* 2012;21(2):172–80.

11. World Health Organization. *Tobacco Industry Interference with Tobacco Control.* Geneva, Switzerland: WHO; 2008.

12. Assunta M. *Global Tobacco Industry Interference Index 2019.* Bangkok, Thailand.

Annexure 1

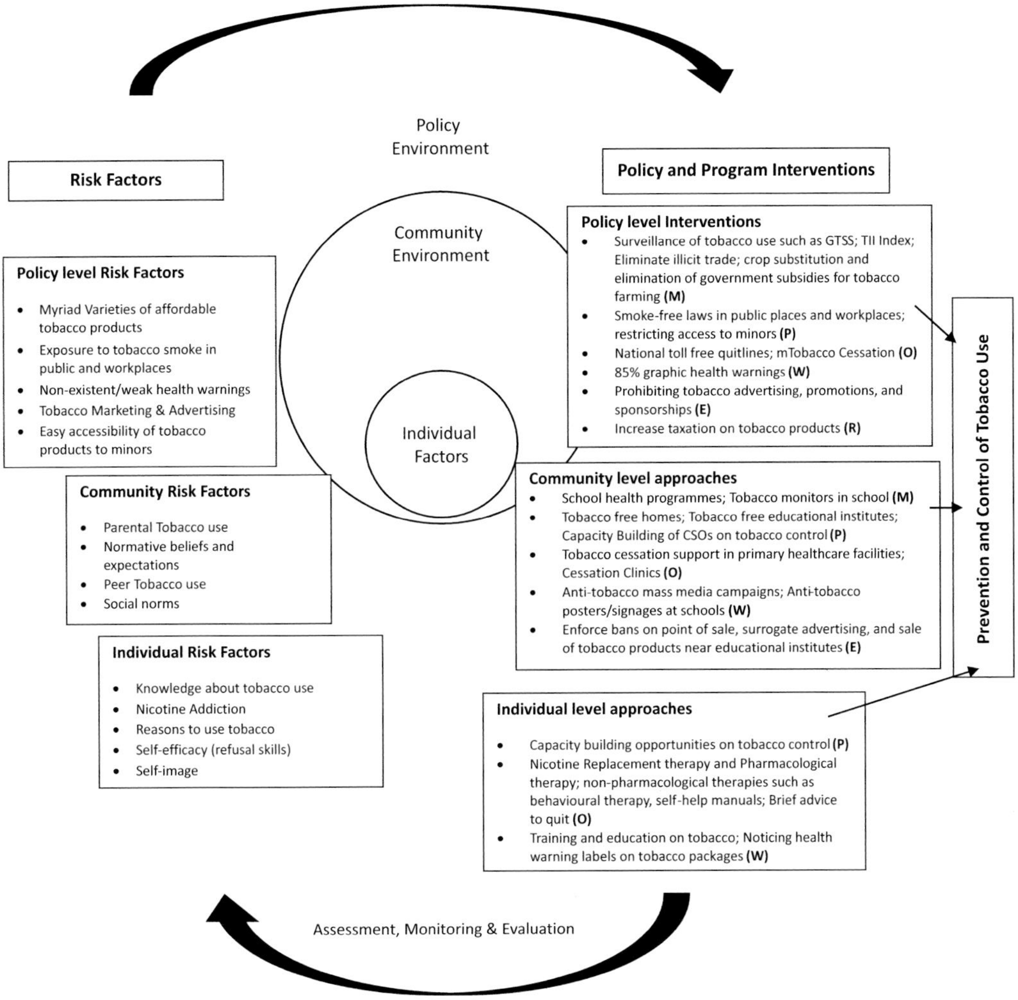

MPOWER

M = Monitor tobacco use and prevention policies

P = Protect people from tobacco smoke

O = Offer help to quit tobacco use

W = Warn about dangers of tobacco

E = Enforce bans of tobacco advertising, promotion, and sponsorship

R = Raise taxes on tobacco

DOI: 10.1201/b23385-12

Case Study: *Sustaining Behavior Change: Institutionalizing Health Interventions*

K.R. Thankappan and G.K. Mini

CONTENTS

QUIT TOBACCO INTERNATIONAL (QTI)

> Project Quit Tobacco International (QTI) developed and implemented tobacco cessation modules for the undergraduate medical curriculum in India and Indonesia.
>
> QTI was successful in incorporating tobacco education in the undergraduate medical curriculum of two health universities in the Kerala and Karnataka states in India.
>
> QTI successfully piloted a community-based smoke-free home initiative in India and Indonesia that was scaled up in both countries.

The QTI project was a pioneering effort started to increase the capacity of tobacco cessation research, training, and practice in India and Indonesia.[1] Three areas were covered under the program:

1. *Modules*: Fifteen modules on tobacco cessation were developed focusing on the public health importance of tobacco control, the relationship between tobacco and specific organ systems, diseases related to smoking and chewing tobacco, and the impact of tobacco on medication effectiveness. Training videos were also developed.
2. *Community outreach, smoke-free homes*[2]: As part of the piloting, a survey was conducted to assess the prevalence of secondhand smoke exposure at the household level after which the intervention program was implemented. The implantation was through Kudumbasree, a large women's organization in Kerala. This program was scaled up across the state by the Kerala Government Health Department. Similar activity was done in Indonesia.[3] The findings indicated that the percentage of smokers who did not smoke inside their homes increased from 11% to 54% in a post-intervention survey.[4]
3. *Randomized controlled trial*: The trial compared the effectiveness of a strong diabetes-specific cessation message delivered by doctors and the added advantage of diabetes-specific cessation counseling by a non-doctor health professional on tobacco quit rates among diabetes patients.[5] The findings indicated that a brief intervention by a doctor resulted in a quit rate of more than 10%. The study demonstrated that the odds of quitting were close to nine times higher for the group that received cessation counseling compared to the group that received a doctor's quit advice only. Similar findings were reported in Indonesia.[6] Quitting or harm reduction in the intervention group was significantly higher compared with the control group at one year.[7]

CONTROL OF HYPERTENSION IN RURAL INDIA

With the aim to estimate the prevalence, awareness, treatment, and control of hypertension and to develop strategies to better manage hypertension in rural communities in India, the Control of Hypertension in Rural India (CHIRI) program was conducted in three diverse rural regions in

 DOI: 10.1201/b23385-13

India: Trivandrum, Kerala; the West Godavari District, Northern Andhra Pradesh; and the Rishi Valley region in Southern Andhra Pradesh.[8]

> Control of Hypertension in Rural India (CHIRI) effectively implemented a feasible community-based intervention for behavioral change to hypertension management in rural India through Accredited Social Health Activists (ASHAs).
>
> CHIRI provides evidence that a low-cost intervention program using ASHAs is effective in controlling blood pressure in low-resource settings.
>
> CHIRI is a potentially scalable model to manage hypertension in low-resource settings.

The CHIRI program developed and implemented a training package for Accredited Social Health Activists (ASHAs) to identify and control hypertension in the community, and evaluated the effectiveness of the training program using the Kirkpatrick Evaluation Model.[9]

In addition to health education, several other components such as improving adherence to antihypertensive medications, encouraging lifestyle changes such as losing excess weight, and increasing physical activity were incorporated into the intervention. We found that this approach resulted in reductions in systolic and diastolic blood pressure (BP) in the intervention group compared to the control group (decline in systolic BP: –5.0 mm Hg, decline in diastolic BP: –2.1 mm Hg). The proportion of those who controlled their hypertension was also found to be greater in the intervention than in the control group in all three regions of the study. This study indicated that group-based intervention, delivered by community health workers for three months, is an efficient way to improve the management of hypertension in diverse rural settings in India that can be applied across rural India to improve cardiovascular health.

KERALA DIABETES PREVENTION PROGRAM

> The Kerala Diabetes Prevention Program (KDPP) was effective in reducing the incidence of diabetes and cardiometabolic risk factors.
>
> KDPP was scaled up in three other districts of Kerala with the help of a large women's organization reaching up to 375,000 individuals.

The Kerala Diabetes Prevention Program (KDPP) is the first cluster randomized controlled trial of a culturally tailored and group-based lifestyle intervention program targeting a rural population at high risk of developing type 2 diabetes mellitus (T2DM) based on a validated risk-assessment questionnaire.[10] The objectives of the program were to (1) evaluate the effectiveness of KDPP on the incidence of T2DM at 24 months; (2) identify the individual, household, and neighborhood-level factors likely to influence the scalability of KDPP in India and other developing countries in the future; and (3) estimate the cost-effectiveness of screening and intervention in reducing the incidence of T2DM.

The findings of KDPP indicated that after a median follow-up of 24 months, T2DM developed in 17.1% of control participants and 14.9% of intervention participants. Compared with the control group, the incidence of type 2 diabetes was reduced by 36% among intervention participants with high program compliance (attended 11–15 sessions). Overall, at 24 months, compared to the control group, intervention participants had a lower decline in HDL cholesterol, a lower increase in the total cholesterol/HDL ratio, a reduction in current alcohol use, a greater increase in fruit and vegetable intake, and an improved physical functioning score of the health-related quality of life index scale. The average cost for providing the peer-support intervention was US$22.50 per participant. The study concluded that a low-cost community-based peer-support lifestyle intervention resulted in a nonsignificant reduction in diabetes incidence in the high-risk population at 24 months, and there was a significant improvement in some cardiovascular disease risk factors and quality of life in the intervention group compared to the control group. Such cost-effective programs offer important opportunities for future implementation of health promotion programs in low- and middle-income settings.

COMMUNITY INTERVENTIONS FOR HEALTH

Community Interventions for Health (CIH) was a pilot study focusing on the prevention of noncommunicable diseases (NCDs) in developing countries.[11] The three settings of the study were Kerala in India, Hangzhou city in China, and Mexico City in Mexico. CIH used multicomponent tailored interventions that were environment friendly and demonstrated that culturally sensitive, community-based interventions for health were feasible and found to be effective in controlling risk factors of NCDs in low- and middle-income countries.

> Community Interventions for Health (CIH) developed culturally appropriate, community-based interventions for reducing noncommunicable disease (NCD) risk factors and implemented them in schools, workplaces, and at the community level in India, China, and Mexico.
>
> CIH demonstrated that health promotion interventions for controlling NCD risk factors are feasible, affordable, and effective in low- and middle-income countries.
>
> Interventions for controlling NCD risk factors need cultural adaptation.

At the community level, two independent cross-sectional surveys among adults aged 18–64 years were conducted at baseline and follow-up. Culturally appropriate interventions were delivered for a period of 18–24 months in the intervention group. CIH used structural interventions and community mobilization that were supported by health education and social marketing. Most of the interventions were planned in such a way that they could be implemented in low-resource settings resulting in significant cost savings. A total of 6194 adults were covered at baseline and 6022 at follow-up in India, China, and Mexico. Overweight significantly increased from 32% to 41% in the control group and there was no such significant change in the intervention group (36% vs. 38%). Tobacco use among men increased in the control group and decreased in the intervention group (change in the control group: 2.7, change in the intervention group: –0.7). There was a reduction in salt intake in both groups, but this decrease was more prominent in the intervention group (change in the control group: –14.0, change in the intervention group: –20.6). A positive impact of the intervention was also seen in the increase in physical activity.

REFERENCES

1. Nichter M, Project Quit Tobacco International Group. "Introducing Tobacco Cessation Training in Developing Countries: An Overview of Project Quit Tobacco International", *Tobacco Control* 15 Supplement 1(2006): 12–17.

2. Nichter M, Nichter M, Padmawati RS, and Ng N. "Developing a Smoke Free Household Initiative: An Indonesian Case Study", *Acta Obstetricia et Gynecologica Scandinavica* 89(2010): 578–81.

3. Padmawati RS, Prabandari YS, Istiyani T, Nichter M, and Nichter M. "Establishing a Community-Based Smoke-Free Homes Movement in Indonesia", *Tobacco Prevention & Cessation* 4(2018): 36.

4. Prabandari YS, Nichter M, Nichter M, Padmawathi RS., and Muramoto M. "Laying the Groundwork for Tobacco Cessation Education in Medical Colleges in Indonesia", *Education for Health (Abingdon, England)* 28(2015): 169–175.

5. Thankappan KR, Mini GK, Daivadanam M, Vijayakumar G, Sarma PS, and Nichter M. "Smoking Cessation among Diabetes Patients: Results of a Pilot Randomized Controlled Trial in Kerala, India", *BMC Public Health* 13(2013): 47.

6. Ng N, Nichter M, Padmawati RS, Prabandari YS, Muramoto M, and Nichter M. "Bringing Smoking Cessation to Diabetes Clinics in Indonesia", *Chronic Illness* 6(2010): 125–135.

7. Thankappan KR, Mini GK, Hariharan M, Vijayakumar G, Sarma PS, and Nichter M. "Smoking Cessation Among Diabetic Patients in Kerala, India: 1-Year Follow-Up Results from a Pilot Randomized Controlled Trial", *Diabetes Care* 37(2014): e256–257.

8. Riddell MA, Joshi R, Oldenburg B, Chow C, et al. "Cluster Randomised Feasibility Trial to Improve the Control of Hypertension in Rural India (CHIRI): A Study Protocol", *BMJ Open* 6(2016): e012404.

9. Abdel-All M, Thrift AG, Riddell M, Thankappan KR, et al. "Evaluation of a Training Program of Hypertension for Accredited Social Health Activists (ASHA) in Rural India", *BMC Health Service Research* 18 (2018): 320.

10. Sathish T, Williams ED, Pasricha N, Absetz P, et al. "Cluster Randomised Controlled Trial of a Peer-Led Lifestyle Intervention Program: Study Protocol for the Kerala Diabetes Prevention Program", *BMC Public Health* 13(2013): 1035.

11. O'Connor Duffany K, Finegood DT, Matthews D, McKee M, et al. "Community Interventions for Health (CIH): A Novel Approach to Tackling the World Wide Epidemic of Chronic Disease", *CVD Prevention and Control* 6(2011): 47–56.

8 Public Health Approaches to Promoting Physical Activity

Gregory W. Heath with contributions by Shifalika Goenka

CONTENTS

> Effective national action to reverse current trends and reduce disparities in physical activity requires a "systems-based" approach with a strategic combination of upstream policy actions aimed at improving the social, cultural, economic and environmental factors that support physical activity, combined with "downstream", individually focused approaches.
>
> **World Health Organization, 2018, "Global Action Plan on Physical Activity 2018–2030: More Active People for a Healthier World"**

INTRODUCTION

Scientific guidelines documenting that regular physical activity (PA) protects against coronary heart disease, type 2 diabetes, some cancers, hypertension, obesity, clinical depression, and other chronic conditions have recently been confirmed by a series of international systematic reviews (Lee et al., 2012, 2018; Guidelines for Physical Activity Scientific Advisory Committee Report, 2018; Powell et al., 2019). In addition, intervention strategies designed to increase physical activity in whole populations are now prominent among contemporary public health initiatives (see Table 8.1). As posited by the ecological model (Sallis et al., 2008), physical activity behaviors are influenced by factors that coexist and interact at multiple levels, which are broadly conceived as personal (i.e., biological and psychological attributes), social (i.e., family, affiliation group, and work influences), and environmental (i.e., contexts for different forms of physical activity as well as policy factors that may determine the availability of relevant settings and opportunities) (Sallis et al., 2008; Global Advocacy for Physical Activity, 2010). Thus, intersectoral approaches that operate at various levels of influence may be more successful in increasing levels of physical activity than those that target only one level (Piercy et al., 2019).

Previous reports have summarized representative evidence-based physical activity interventions from across the globe that were linked to a broad understanding of health promotion and disease prevention at national, state/regional, and local levels (Heath et al., 2012; Sallis et al., 2016). In such a 'review of reviews,' there has been a paucity of studies identified that evaluate community-based physical activity strategies among low- to middle-income countries (LMICs). Therefore, this chapter seeks to update physical activity interventions consisting of a primary and secondary search of the literature, focusing on studies and reviews representative of effective and promising physical activity interventions carried out among LMICs from around the world. We searched the English, Spanish, and Portuguese literature using the same search methods as reported in the initial reports, including the LILACS database to specifically search the Spanish and Portuguese literature (Sallis et al., 2016). A table is provided summarizing the previous search results including more recent published studies. These reviews and original studies are listed by lead author, setting (e.g., school, worksite, community, and health care), countries represented, population

 DOI: 10.1201/b23385-14

Table 8.1: Summary of Physical Activity Intervention Studies Reviewed

	Campaigns and Informational Approaches/ Community-Wide Campaigns	Behavioral and Social	Policy and Environmental/Community-Wide Policies and Planning
Number of studies included	5	9	1
Summary of Studies Included by Intervention Domain/Strategy			
Countries Represented	Iran, China, South Africa, India, Indonesia, Vietnam	Vanuatu, India, South Africa, Chile, Brazil, China, Pakistan	Colombia
% (#) of studies with some evidence	80 (4/5)	56 (5/9)	100 (1/1)

Characteristics of Studies Included by Intervention Domain/Strategy

Author (Year)	Study Period	Study Design	Country	Intervention Strategy	Study Population/ Setting Description	Sample Size	Results: Effect Measure	Results: Value Used in Summary	Follow-Up Time
Campaigns and Informational Approaches/Community-Wide Campaigns									
Rabiei (2010)	2000–2006	QE[1]	Iran	Education – public media and campaigns for entire population and specific target groups; Environment – urban environment modifications to reduce personal vehicle use and promote active transportation (e.g., cycling) Policy – adding exercise time in the afternoon shift of schools	Adult residents of 3 communities in central Iran (intervention areas: 1 urban, 1 rural; reference area: 1 urban/rural)	Baseline N = 6000 (Intervention/ reference *n* not reported)	Δ LTPA and Transportation PA	Δ LTPA (MET-min/d), 2001 vs. 2000 Women I = +13.4*; R = +6.5* Men I = +7.3***; R = −10.9 Δ Transportation PA (MET-min/d), 2001 vs. 2000 Women I = −3.3; R = −30.9* Men I = −12.4; R = −46.7*	2 years
Lv (2014)	2008–2011	QE[1]	China	Community mobilization, structural change, health education, social marketing	Adult residents of 3 adjacent districts of Hangzhou, China (2 intervention; 1 reference area)	Baseline I = 1016 R = 1000	Δ reported total PA (walking, moderate PA, and vigorous PA)	Δ PA (MET-min/wk) I – sig Δ in low levels of PA, no Δ in R sites Sig Δ in mod PA and vig PA in I and decrease in R sites Total PA net Δ of +5% in I sites vs. R sites	2 years

(Continued)

Table 8.1 (Continued): Summary of Physical Activity Intervention Studies Reviewed

Campaigns and Informational Approaches/ Community-Wide Campaigns									
Behavioral and Social									
Policy and Environmental/Community-Wide Policies and Planning									
Krishnan (2011)	2003–2008	CS[3]	India and Indonesia	Media; environmental change; health messages	Adult residents of 2 selected sites: 1 in India and 1in Indonesia	Baseline India N = 5143 Indonesia N = 1806	Work, leisure time, and transportation PA	Δ Inactivity (%) India Men: –3.0; Women: +18.3*** Indonesia Men: –3.9; Women: –19.2***	3 years
Nguyen (2012)	2006–2009	QE[1]	Viet Nam	Media; health messages; community support	Adult residents of two rural communes (1 intervention; 1 reference)	I = 2,298 R = 2352	Work, leisure-time, and transportation PA	Δ Physical inactivity (%) I vs. R +6.1 net effect – (I site underwent rapid urban change vs. R community)	3 years
Behavioral and Social									
Siefken (2015)	2011	CS[3]	Vanuatu	Health messages; walking campaign	Female civil servants at one worksite	N = 207	Pedometer measured steps over 12 weeks	Net increase in steps – pre-post = +26% among all subjects Net steps low risk (n = 101) +82%; high risk (n = 24), 228%	12 weeks
Kain (2014)	2011–2012	RT[4]	Chile	Classroom nutrition education; increase physical education (PE) class time; increase time in moderate activity during PE classes	6–8 y/o low-income students attending primary school in Santiago – exposed or not exposed to intervention	I = 651 C = 823	Δ PE class time Δ class time in MVPA as measured by pedometer	Δ PE class time (min) I = +9.1 C = +3.4 Δ Class time in MVPA (%) I = –1.1 C = –8.3*	1 year
Balagopal (2012)	2007–2008	CS[3]	India	Community health worker (CHW)-delivered health education; social support	Adult residents of selected rural community; low and high SES	N = 1638	Work PA; household chores; brisk walking; vigorous or manual PA; transportation PA; leisure-time PA	Δ MVPA (%): +11.6** among normal fasting blood glucose participants; +14.2** among glucose intolerant; +4.2*** among T2DM participants	6 months

(Continued)

Table 8.1 (Continued): Summary of Physical Activity Intervention Studies Reviewed

			Campaigns and Informational Approaches/ Community-Wide Campaigns		Behavioral and Social		Policy and Environmental/Community-Wide Policies and Planning		
Skaal (2012)	2008	QE[1]	South Africa	Social support; media; PA challenge	Hospital employees (medical and nonmedical)	Medical n = 100; Non-medical n = 100	Self-report stage of physical activity based on transtheoretical model (TTM)	TTM mean stages Pre-test = 2.64 Post-test = 3.74***	6 months
Vio (2011)	2006	QE[1]	Chile	PA classes led by trained instructors 3×/week for 6 months	Low SES women residing in selected community 4 groups: GrA – PA; GrB – diet only; GrC – PA; GrD – control	N = 331 GrA = 82 GrB = 80 GrC = 84 GrD = 85	PA class adherence	Mean PA class adherence: GrA = 49.8%; GrC = 37.5%	6 months
Parra (2010)	2007	CS[3]	Brazil	PA classes (*Academia da Cidade* – ACP) in public parks led by PA instructors	Community residents of Recife who visited both ACP and non-ACP parks	32,974 people (adults/ children/youth) observed during 5589 observation visits to ACP and non-ACP parks	PA Observed - SOPARC among people visiting both ACP and non-ACP parks	People using ACP parks more likely to engage in MVPA (64% vs. 49%) More women (45% vs. 42%) and older adults (14.7% vs. 5.7%) in ACP vs. non-ACP sites	5 years
Mendonca (2010)	2008	CS[3]	Brazil	PA classes (*Academia da Cidade* – ACP) in public parks led by PA instructors	Adult residents of selected community	N = 2267	Meeting PA guidelines based on leisure-time MVPA	Meeting guidelines was associated with having ever heard about ACP [OR 1.8 (95% CI: 1.4, 2.2)]; having seen a ACP class [OR = 1.6 (95% CI: 1.1, 2.3)]; being a current ACP participant [OR = 14.3 (95% CI: 12.3,16.4)]; and being a past ACP participant [OR = 4.0 (95% CI: 1.4, 11.3)]	4 years

(*Continued*)

Table 8.1 (Continued): Summary of Physical Activity Intervention Studies Reviewed

Campaigns and Informational Approaches/ Community-Wide Campaigns									
Behavioral and Social									
Policy and Environmental/Community-Wide Policies and Planning									
Li (2011)	2009	QE[1]	China	Classroom-based PA sessions: 2 daily 10-min PA sessions in between class breaks (Happy10 program)	8–11 y/o students attending primary schools in Beijing – exposed or not exposed to Happy10	N = 4700	Self-report PA – 7 day recall; BMI z-scores	Mean Δ in BMI z-scores between I schools vs. R schools = −0.15 kg/m^2 Post 1** and 2*** year = I maintained BMI z vs. R schools	2 years
Almas (2013)	2008	QE[1]	Pakistan	School-based PE program 30 min sessions, 4×/wk	9–11 y/o school girls from 4 schools (2 Intervention; 2 Reference)	I = 131 R = 146	Adherence to PE classes; Reported PA	I adherence = 80%; R adherence = 78.5% No net difference in reported PA	20 weeks
Jemmont (2014)	2007–2010	RT[4]	South Africa	Small group activities, games, brainstorming, videos, discussions	Men reporting coitus in the previous 3 months and living in one of the selected neighborhoods randomized to condition (PA vs. attention-control)	I = 572 C = 609	Adherence to PA guidelines by self-report	% Meeting PA guidelines Total PA OR – I vs. C = 1.28 (1.05, 1.57); PA vig – 1.30 (1.06, 1.57); PA mod – OR 1.25(1.02, 1.52)	1 year
Policy and Environmental/Community-Wide Policies and Planning									
Torres (2013)	2009	CS[3]	Colombia	Community planning and policies – Ciclovia (public streets) and Cicloruta (bike paths)	Adult residents of selected community	Ciclovia N = 1000 Cicloruta N = 1000	Meeting PA guidelines	Meeting PA guidelines among regular participants vs. infrequent participants of Ciclovia – OR = 1.7 (1.1, 2.4) Meeting PA guidelines among regular users vs. infrequent users of Cicloruta – OR = 10.2 (6.1, 16.8)	N/A

[1] *Quasi-experimental – intervention and referent communities/sites*
[2] *Cohort – pre-intervention and post-intervention measures*
[3] *Cross-sectional – pre–post-intervention measures*
[4] *Randomized prospective study – intervention vs. control group*
[5] *Other*
* $p < 0.0001$, ** $p < 0.01$, *** $p < 0.05$

characteristics, intervention domain/strategy, outcome measures used, assessment of effectiveness, and period of follow-up (Heath et al., 2012; Sallis et al., 2016) (see Table 8.1).

The intervention strategies were classified using the domains established by the Guide to Community Preventive Services (*The Community Guide*; Kahn et al., 2005). These domains are used to conveniently capture most physical activity intervention strategies delivered throughout the world and consist of descriptors that are found in other international physical activity recommendation documents including The Lancet Physical Activity Series (LPAS) (World Health Organization, 2010; Heath et al., 2012; Sallis et al., 2016; Ding et al., 2019).

These intervention strategy domains include:

1. *Campaigns and informational approaches*, which target changing knowledge, attitudes, and behavior about the benefits of and opportunities for physical activity within a community.
2. *Behavioral and social approaches*, which consist of teaching people the behavioral management skills that are necessary for successful adoption and maintenance of behavior change, and working through or creating organizational and social environments that facilitate and enhance behavioral change.
3. *Environmental and policy approaches*, which are aimed at structuring the physical and organizational environments so that people have accessible, safe, attractive, and convenient places to be physically active (see Table 8.2).

Strategies from each intervention domain were selected from a series of original reviews (van de Vijvera et al., 2012; Hoehner et al., 2013; Bull et al., 2014; Baker et al., 2015) that demonstrated a net intervention effect as part of an original study; represented at least one of the three intervention domains; a study of children, youth, or adult subjects without established disease; provision of a detailed study protocol; availability of a physical activity outcome measure; and a study duration of three months or longer (Roux et al., 2008).

PHYSICAL ACTIVITY INTERVENTIONS THAT WORK IN LMICS

Campaigns and Informational Approaches

Community-Wide Campaigns

A recommended strategy within this intervention domain is community-wide campaigns, which often employ multicomponent (e.g., use of media, behavioral, social, policy, and environmental

Table 8.2: Overview of Strategies to Promote Physical Activity in Communities

Approach	Strategy	Classification
Campaigns and informational	Point-of-decision prompts	Effective
	Community-wide campaigns	Effective
	Mass media campaigns	Promising
	Short informational messages	Promising
Behavioral and social	School-based strategies – physical education	Effective
	Social support in communities	Effective
	Family-based physical activity	Effective
	Combined diet and physical activity promotion programs to prevent type 2 diabetes among people at increased risk	Effective
	Physical activity interventions that include activity monitors for overweight or obese adults	Effective
	Physical activity digital health interventions for adults 55 years and older	Effective
	Provider-based assessment and counseling	Promising
	Community physical activity classes	Promising
Policy and environmental	Physical activity: built environment approaches combining transportation system interventions with land use and environmental design	Effective
	Creating or improving places for physical activity	Effective
	Interventions to increase active travel to school	Effective
	Community-wide planning and policies	Promising

Sources: https://www.thecommunityguide.org/topic/physical-activity; Heath et al., *Lancet* 2012; 380:272–81; Sallis et al., *Lancet* 2016 Sep 24;388(10051):1325–36.

approaches), multisector, and multisite interventions (Heath et al., 2012). These campaigns represent large-scale, high-intensity, high-visibility programming and often use TV, radio, newspapers, and other media to raise program awareness, disseminate targeted/segmented health messages, and reinforce behavior change. Community-wide interventions from the current body of evidence among LMICs include the cardiovascular disease prevention program in Iran (Rabiei et al., 2010), where the interventions included a campaign with media and health education programming for noncommunicable disease (NCD) prevention through physical activity along with provider-based counseling, community groups, active transport promotion, and physical activity programming within neighborhood park spaces. The intervention period lasted two years and was carried out in two Iranian urban centers, one large and one medium, compared to a referent community of similar size. Changes in leisure-time physical activity were documented among both men and women in the intervention communities with a net intervention effect compared to the referent community of 7% and 17% among women and men, respectively (Rabiei et al., 2010). Other community-wide campaign interventions reviewed include the Hangzhou District's (China) health promotion program (Lv et al., 2014); a South African physical activity promotion program (Jemmont et al., 2014); a health promotion campaign in Viet Nam (Nguyen et al., 2012); and NCD prevention trials in India and Indonesia (Krishnan et al., 2010) (see Table 8.1). These studies, mostly using a quasi-experimental design, contrast with the initial LPAS review, which showed the majority of studies among LMICs were observational studies or studies with insufficient evidence. Those with insufficient evidence were not necessarily ineffective but showed inconsistent evidence in support of community-wide interventions (Heath et al., 2012; Sallis et al., 2016). Therefore, the body of evidence for community-wide campaigns appears to be growing in volume and quality among LMICs since the initial LPAS reviews (Heath et al.; Sallis et al., 2016).

Behavioral and Social Approaches

Social Support Interventions in Community Settings

Social support in community settings is an example of a strategy that capitalizes on existing social networks to reinforce physical activity behavior. Behavioral and social approaches include creating buddy systems, contracting, and forming walking or other physical activity support groups. An exemplary intervention that represents this strategy, as reported by Balagopal et al. (2012), is one in which men and women from local communities within a larger urban area in India were organized into physical activity groups within their neighborhoods and received communications (e.g., health education brochures and individual visits) by trained community health workers. The intervention was designed to reinforce and sustain the participants' physical activity social network. Other examples of physical activity interventions that utilized social support/networking include the work of Skaal and Pengpid (2012) in South Africa among healthcare workers; and among female civil servants in Vanuatu, an isolated South Pacific Island (Siefken et al., 2014).

Physical Activity Classes in Community Settings

Evidence of the effectiveness of community-wide physical activity programs is still emerging, as shown by the promising impact of providing physical activity classes at the community level to increase physical activity levels. These programs offer fitness instruction and aerobics classes for the population at no charge to the participants and are often carried out in public places (e.g., parks, school yards, community centers, worksites, and common sports facilities). Parra et al. (2010) assessed park use in Recife, Brazil, examining the differences in physical activity rates comparing parks with and without the Academia da Cidade Program (ACP; physical activity classes in public parks), where people using ACP parks were more likely to be seen engaging in both moderate and vigorous aerobic physical activity compared to non-ACP park users. Mendonca et al. (2010) showed similar results where ACP park users in Aracaju, Brazil, were at an odds of 1.8 of achieving recommended levels of physical activity (150 minutes per week) compared with non-ACP park users. Vio et al. (2011) provide evidence of improved attendance and adherence to such programs regardless of socioeconomic status and location of the classes among low-income women in Santiago, Chile.

School-Based Interventions

A recommended strategy within the behavioral and social domain is school-based physical education (PE). School-based interventions have great potential to increase levels of physical activity among children because in many countries PE is mandatory, which increases participation even among the least active children. School-based interventions include programs delivered during school time as well as after school (Heath et al., 2012). The effects of school-based interventions have been evaluated using various outcomes such as physical activity level, fitness, obesity, other cardiovascular risk factors, and well-being. Three school-based physical activity intervention studies representing LMICs have been identified (Almas et al., 2013; Li et al., 2010; Kain et al., 2014) as well as one recent systematic review of school-based physical activity promotion among adolescents representing 63 LMICs (Peralta et al., 2020). Almas et al. (2013) carried out a school-based intervention among local schoolgirls in Karachi, Pakistan, and demonstrated good adherence to the sessions by the girls. However, measured physical activity did not show statistically significant changes compared to the control schools where the intervention was not delivered. Nevertheless, Li et al. (2010) demonstrated the effectiveness of classroom physical activity interventions among students in Beijing, China, schools over one and two years, reporting that the intervention group was more likely to maintain their body mass index (BMI) z-scores compared to the control groups where BMI increased. Kain et al. (2014) carried out a school-based obesity prevention program among six- to eight-year-old low-income children in Chile. Nutrition education classes coupled with increased physical education frequency and duration of sessions to include increased moderate to vigorous physical activity comprised the intervention. Referent schools without the enhanced intervention were compared with intervention schools. There was a significant net increase in physical activity time during school comparing the intervention and referent schools. Children exposed to the intervention were at lesser odds of increasing their BMI over the study period compared with children not exposed to the intervention (Kain et al., 2014).

Policy and Environmental Approaches

Community-Wide Policies and Programs

This potentially effective intervention strategy characterized by using community-wide policies and planning combined with multicomponent efforts at the community level has been implemented in Latin America to promote physical activity (Heath et al., 2012; Sallis et al., 2016; Guide to Community Preventive Services, 2020). These community action plans and policies are designed to reduce environmental and structural barriers (e.g., the lack of bike lanes/paths and proximity to vehicular traffic) that directly impact physical activity behaviors. Plans and policies are promoted through media campaigns and incentives at various levels (e.g., individual, corporate, local, and regional). This type of intervention strategy not only provides information that is intended to motivate individual behavior change, but also focuses on providing institutional and environmental (i.e., structural, social, and cultural) support to sustain physical activity behavior change over time (Heath et al., 2012; Sallis et al., 2016; Ding et al., 2019). Torres et al. (2013) reported that respondents to community surveys assessing the level of participation in such intervention strategies in Colombia demonstrated greater odds of achieving physical activity guidelines when participation was reported to be regular (i.e., four or more days per month), with regular Ciclovia participants with a 1.7 odds ratio of achieving physical activity guidelines and regular Cicloruta participants (five to seven days per week) being ten times more likely compared with infrequent participants in these intervention strategies, respectively.

PROMOTING PHYSICAL ACTIVITY IN COMMUNITIES: LIMITATIONS AND NEXT STEPS

Several limitations are associated with the present review. Although an attempt was made to canvas the global literature irrespective of language, the current review draws primarily from the published literature representing the languages of English, Spanish, and Portuguese. Also, there was no attempt to complete a search of the gray literature, and a significant portion of the literature reviewed lacked measures of external validity and hence limited the generalizability of the findings to other settings and countries. Despite these limitations, these findings should be valuable to LMIC practitioners as well as physical activity and health scientists.

Hence, based on the aforementioned findings, there is a significant number of evidence-based approaches that demonstrate an acceptable level of effectiveness that have been implemented over the past four to five years among LMICs. However, further documentation of the adaptation, tailoring, and evaluation of current physical activity interventions among LMICs needs broader dissemination, especially since NCDs have become a primary public health challenge among these countries.

CONFLICTS OF INTEREST

We declare that we have no conflicts of interest. The findings and conclusions in this report are those of the authors and do not necessarily represent the official position of any of the organizations, institutions, or agencies to which they are affiliated.

ACKNOWLEDGMENTS

The author wishes to acknowledge the co-authors and executive committee of The Lancet Physical Activity Series for their collegial support and feedback in the development of this chapter.

REFERENCES

Physical Activity Guidelines Advisory Committee. *Physical Activity Guidelines Advisory Committee Scientific Report.* Washington, DC: US Department of Health and Human Services; 2018.

Almas A, Islam M, Jafar TH. School-based physical activity programme in preadolescent girls (9–11 years): A feasibility trial in Karachi, Pakistan. *Arch Diseases in Children.* 2013;98:515–519.

Baker PRA, Francis DP, Soares J, Weightman AL, Foster C. Community wide interventions for increasing physical activity. *Cochrane Database Syst Rev.* 2015(1):CD008366. doi: 10.1002/14651858.CD008366.pub3.

Balagopal P, Patel TG, Misra R. A community-based participatory diabetes prevention and management intervention in rural India using community health workers. *Diabetes Educator.* 2012;38(6):822–834.

Bauman AE, Reis R, Sallis JF, Wells J, Loos R, Martin BW. Correlates of physical activity: Why are some people physically active and others not? *Lancet.* 2012;380:258–71.

Bull ER, Dombrowski SU, McCleary N, et al. Are interventions for low-income groups effective in changing healthy eating, physical activity and smoking behaviours? A systematic review and meta-analysis. *BMJ Open* 2014;4:e006046. doi:10.1136/bmjopen-2014-006046.

Community Preventive Services Task Force. *The Guide to Community Preventive Services: Physical Activity: Built Environment Approaches Combining Transportation System Interventions with Land Use and Environmental Design.* 2016. Available from: http://thecommunityguide.org. Accessed 11/2/2017.

Ding D, Ramirez Varela A, Bauman AE, Ekelund U, Lee IM, Heath GW, et al. Towards better evidence-informed global action: Lessons learnt from the Lancet series and recent developments in physical activity and public health. *Br J Sports Med.* 2019. https://doi.org/10.1136/bjsports-2019-101001.

European Union Sport and Health Working Group. *European Union physical activity guidelines.* Brussels, Belgium: European Union; 2008.

Global Advocacy Council for Physical Activity, International Society for Physical Activity and Health. The Toronto Charter for Physical Activity: A Global Call to Action, J Phys Act Health. 2010 Nov;7 Suppl 3: S370–85. English, Multiple languages. doi: 10.1123/jpah.7.s3.s370. PMID: 21116016.

Guthold R, Stevens GA, Riley LM, Bull FC. Worldwide trends in insufficient physical activity from 2001 to 2016: A pooled analysis of 358 population-based surveys with 1.9 million participants. *Lancet Global Health.* 2018;6(10):e1077–e86.

Heath GW, Brownson RC, Kruger J, Miles R, Powell KE, Ramsey LT. The effectiveness of urban design and land use and transport policies and practices to increase physical activity: A systematic review. *J Phys Act Health.* 2006; 1:S55–S71.

Heath GW, Parra DC, Sarmiento OL, Andersen LB, Owen N, Goenka S, Montes F, Brownson RC. Evidence-based intervention in physical activity: Lessons from around the world. *Lancet* 2012; 380:272–81.

Hoehner CM, Ribeiro IC, Parra DC, Reis RS, Azevedo MR, Hino AA, Soares J, Hallal PC, Simões EJ, Brownson RC. Physical activity interventions in Latin America expanding and classifying the evidence. *Am J Prev Med* 2013;44(3):e31–e40.

Jemmont JB, Jemmont LS, Ngwane Z, et al. Theory-based behavioral intervention increases self-reported physical activity in South African men: A cluster-randomized controlled trial. *Prevent Med.* 2014;64:114–120.

Kahn EB, Ramsey LT, Brownson RC, Heath GW, Howze EH, Powell KE, Stone EJ. Chapter 2, Physical activity. In: *The Guide to Community Preventive Services: What Works to Promote Health.* Zaza S, Briss PA, Harris KW (eds). Oxford University Press, 2005.

Kahn EB, Ramsey LT, Brownson RC, Heath GW, Howze EH, Powell KE, Stone EJ, Rajab MW, Corso P. The effectiveness of interventions to increase physical activity: A systematic review. *Am J Prevent Med.* 2002;22(4S) Supplement:73–107.

Kain J, Concha F, Moreno L, Leyton, B. School-based obesity prevention intervention in Chilean children: Effective in controlling, but not reducing obesity. *J Obes.* 2014;2014:618293;doi:10.1155/2014/618293. Epub 2014 Apr 27.

Krishnan A, Ekowati R, Baridalyne N, Kusumawardani N, Suhardi S, Kapoor SK, Leowski J. Evaluation of community-based interventions for non-communicable diseases: Experiences from India and Indonesia. *Health Promotion Int.* 2010;26(3):276–289.

Lee IM, Shiroma EJ, Lobelo F, Puska P, Blair SN, Katzmarzyk PT. Impact of physical inactivity on the world's major non-communicable diseases. *The Lancet.* 2012;380:219–29.

Li YP, Hu XQ, Schouten EG, Liu AL, Du SM, Li LZ, Cui ZH, Wang D, Kok FJ, Hu FB, Ma GS. Report on childhood obesity in China: Effects and sustainability of physical activity intervention on body composition of Chinese youth. *Biomed Environ Sci.* 2010;23(3):180–187.

Lv J, Liu Q-M, Ren Y-J, He P-P, Wang S-F, Gao F, Li L-M, et al. A community-based multi-level intervention for smoking, physical activity, and diet: Short-term findings from the Community Interventions for Health programme in Hangzhou, China. *J Epidemiol Commun Health.* 2014;68:333–339.

Mendonca BC, Oliveira AC, Toscano JJO, Knuth AG, Borges TT, Lalta DC, Cruz DK, Hallal PC. Exposure to a community-wide physical activity promotion program and leisure-time physical activity in Aracaju, Brazil. *J Phys Act Health.* 2010;7(Suppl 2):S223–S228.

Nguyen AN, Pham ST, Nguyen VL, Weinehall L, Wall S, Bonita R, Byass P. Effectiveness of community-based comprehensive health lifestyle promotion on cardiovascular disease risk factors in a rural Vietnamese population: A quasi-experimental study. *Cardiovasc Dis.* 2012;12:56–66.

Parra DC, McKenzie TL, Ribeiro IC, Hino AAF, Dreisinger M, Coniglio K, Munk M, Brownson RC, Pratt M, Hoehner CM. Assessing physical activity in public parks in Brazil using systematic observation. *Am J Pub Health.* 2010;100:1420–1426.

Peralta M, Henriques-Neto D, Bordado J, Loureiro N, Diz J, and Adilson M. Active commuting to school and physical activity levels among 11 to 16 year-old adolescents from 63 low- and middle-income countries. *Int J Environ Res Public Health.* 2020;17:1276. doi:10.3390/ijerph17041276

Piercy KL, Troiano RP, Ballard RM, Carlson SA, Fulton JE, Galuska DA, George SM, Olson RD. The physical activity guidelines for Americans. *JAMA* (2018) Nov 20;320(19):2020–2028.

Powell KE, King AC, Buchner DM, et al. The scientific foundation for the physical activity guidelines for Americans, 2nd edition. *J Phys Act Health.* 2019;16:1–11.

Rabiei K, Kelishadi R, Srrafzadegan N, Sadri G, Amani A. Short-term results of community-based interventions for improving physical activity: Isfahan Healthy Heart Programme. *Arch Med Sci.* 2010;6(1):32–39.

Ramirez Varela A, Pratt M, Powell K, Lee IM, Bauman A, Heath GW, Martins RC, Kohl H, Hallal PC. worldwide surveillance, policy and research on physical activity and health: The global observatory for physical activity: GoPA! *J Phys Act Health.* 2017 Sep 1;14(9):701–9.

Roux L, Pratt M, Tengs TO, Yore MM, Yanagawa TL, Van Den Bos J, Rutt C, Brownson RC, Powell KE, Heath G, Kohl HW3rd, Teutsch S, Cawley J, Lee IM, West L, Buchner DM. Cost effectiveness of community-based physical activity interventions. *Am J Prevent Med.* 2008;35(6):578–88.

Sallis JF, Bull F, Guthold R, Heath GW, et al. Physical activity 2016: Progress and challenges: Progress in physical activity over the Olympic quadrennium. *Lancet.* 2016 Sep 24;388(10051):1325–36.

Sallis JF, Owen N, and Fisher EB. Ecological models of health behavior. In K. Glanz, B. K. Rimer and K. Viswanath (Eds.), *Health Behavior and Health Education: Theory, Research, and Practice* (pp. 465 –482). Fourth Edition, San Francisco: Jossey-Bass; 2008.

Skaal L, Pengpid S. The predictive validity and effects of using the transtheoretical model to increase the physical activity of healthcare workers in a public hospital in South Africa. *TBM.* 2012;2:384–391.

Siefken K, Schofield G, Schulenkorf N. Process evaluation of a walking programme delivered through the workplace in the South Pacific island of Vanuatu. *Global Health Promotion.* 2014;3(2):1–12.

Torres A, Sarmiento OL, Stuaber C, Zarama R. The Ciclovia and Cicloruta programs: Promising interventions to promote physical activity and social capital in Bogota, Colombia. *Am J Public Health.* 2013;103e:e23–230.

van de Vijvera S, Otia S, Addoc J, de Graft-Aikins A, and Agyemang C. Review of community-based interventions for prevention of cardiovascular diseases in low- and middle-income countries. *Ethn Health.* 2012;17(6):651–676.

Vio F, Lera L, Zaracia I. Evaluación de un programa de intervención nutricional y de actividad física dirigido a mujeres chilenas de bajo nivel socioeconomic [Evaluation of a nutrition and physical activity intervention for Chilean women of low socioeconomic status]. *Arch. Latinoam. Nutr.* 2011;61(4):406–413.

World Health Organization. *Global Recommendations on Physical Activity for Health.* Geneva, Switzerland: WHO Press; 2010.

9 Public Health Approaches to Safe Food and Water

Eram Rao, Sunetra Roday, and Archana Singh

CONTENTS

> Innovations that are guided by smallholder farmers, adapted to local circumstances, and sustainable for the economy and environment will be necessary to ensure food security in the future.
>
> **Bill Gates**

INTRODUCTION

Food and drinking water represent fundamental human needs and access to them constitutes a basic human right. Today, the world produces enough food to feed everyone, but unfortunately, an important part of this food is not safe or healthy, and a large percentage is wasted.

The Present Scenario

With an estimated 600 million cases of foodborne illnesses annually, unsafe food is a threat to human health and economies globally. A multitude of hazards such as pathogens, chemicals, and extraneous objects can cause foodborne illnesses. Recent food safety concerns also include foods that are produced using novel and untested technologies such as genetically modified foods, since consumption of these foods could result in potential adverse health effects in the long run. Typically, food is deemed safe when it does not contain harmful pathogens, chemical residues, drug residues, growth hormone residues, or any other substance that could pose health risks (Wang, 2018).

Low- and middle-income countries (LMICs) in general and India as well face a huge burden of unsafe food and unsafe water. High-income countries (HICs) have been able to ensure safe food and water through systems of strong regulation, implementation, and monitoring. In India, the problem is further magnified as a large proportion of food is sold on the streets in open carts or stalls, often located in filthy surroundings near sources of contamination. Unlicensed and licensed food vendors, operating in compromised conditions, with severe financial constraints and without access to even safe drinking water end up serving unsafe food and water to consumers. A partial reason could be ignorance. But in the larger game of things, even consumers may not have a choice even if they are aware due to financial and availability issues. Very often food is wrapped in newspaper, or hot food and beverages in plastic bags and served risking printing ink in the food and plastic leaching into hot food.

There is no food security without food safety. Access to safe food is a central element of public health and is fundamental to the 2030 Agenda for Sustainable Development Goals. Without food safety, we cannot eradicate hunger and malnutrition or achieve healthy lives for all. LMICs need to address this in a very important way.

DOI: 10.1201/b23385-15

From a planetary approach, a food system and health promotion approach that ensures optimal health and well-being for our planet is also important. An integrated approach – one that involves the whole of society – can provide effective and equitable solutions to our contemporary challenges.

Health Promotion and Food Safety

The three pillars of health promotion are (1) good governance, (2) health literacy, and (3) healthy cities. Safe food is a basic foundation on which healthy food can be built upon.

The Eat Right India movement is a food safety and health promotion initiative that adopts a whole-government approach to ensure that policies and programs across the line ministries are synergized together. The key objective is to ensure that every Indian has access to safe, healthy, and sustainable food. Effective food safety and quality control systems are key not only to safeguarding the health and well-being of people, but also to fostering economic development and improving livelihoods by promoting access to domestic, regional, and international markets.

FOOD SAFETY ISSUES IN THE FOOD SUPPLY CHAIN

The Food Safety Context

An emerging economy like India requires safe food to fuel a healthy, educated, and resilient workforce. Foodborne diseases impede socioeconomic development by straining healthcare systems, and harming national economies, tourism, and trade.

Unsafe food contains microbiological, chemical, or physical hazards that can make people sick, causing acute or chronic illness that in extreme cases lead to death or permanent disability. Therefore, it is necessary to understand the different types of food hazards, their entry points into the food chain, and ways to reduce our exposure to these hazards. Consumption of unsafe food also reduces the bioavailability of nutrients, particularly for vulnerable populations. Further, the presence of food safety hazards can lead to food losses and reduce availability for food-insecure populations.

A study recently conducted on foodborne disease in India predicts that the prevalence of foodborne disease will rise from 100 million cases in 2011 to 150 million–177 million cases by 2030 in a business-as-usual scenario (FSSAI, 2020; India Food Vision, 2020).

Food Safety Implementation from 'Farm to Fork'

There is a need to adopt a food system approach to food safety that focuses on the entire value chain and the wider environment in which the chain operates. This farm-to-fork approach recognizes that food can become contaminated at various stages of the value chain and, likewise, that corrective actions should be taken at multiple stages of the chain. The adoption of good agricultural practices (GAP), good hygiene practices (GHP), and good manufacturing practices (GMP) in the entire value chain helps to keep food safe.

As part of enhancing food safety management capacity, it is, therefore, necessary to locate and deal with the weak stages of agri-food value chains, and to build in controls often at multiple levels of the chain to ensure food safety at the point of consumption (Figure 9.1). The primary emphasis, however, should be on avoiding hazards from entering the agri-food chain in the first place (for example, from soil, water, animals, production inputs, and food handlers), and building in ways to detect, remove, and neutralize hazards that occur. Some food safety risks can best be managed at the preharvest stage, for example, antimicrobial residues in animal source foods or pesticide residues in fresh fruit and vegetables. Other food safety risks may need actions at multiple stages of the value chain, such as foods that undergo significant processing between production to consumption.

A broad range of initiatives are being carried out in India to strengthen the contributions that consumers can make to better food safety outcomes. In 2017, the Food Safety and Standards Authority of India (FSSAI) launched an interactive educational online portal to convert 'all food purchasers into smart, alert and aware consumers.' The portal uses food safety display boards showing practices that food business operators must follow, and provides contacts for consumers to provide feedback, queries, and complaints.

To spread its food safety message, the WHO published the manual *Five Keys to Safer Food* for use by health professionals. The manual includes five core messages for safer food: keep clean, separate raw and cooked, cook thoroughly, keep food at safe temperatures, and use safe water and raw materials.

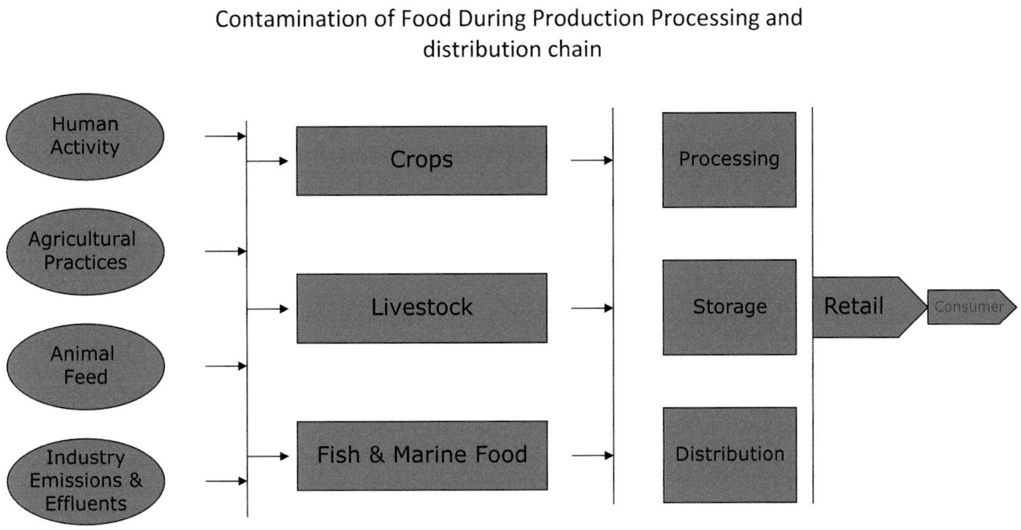

Figure 9.1 Contamination of food during the production, processing, and distribution chain.

APPROACHES TO SAFE, SUSTAINABLE FOOD AND WATER

Strategies for Safe Food and Clean Water

The future of food safety lies in establishing a stringent monitoring evaluation and accountability mechanism in food and water safety. Unfortunately, efforts to strengthen food safety systems remain fragmented and the gains are well below expectations (WHO International Food Safety Conference 2019).

Ensuring that every food business operator has a license or registration (depending on the volume of business) with the FSSAI to carry on a food business in India is the first step. A robust enforcement mechanism should be in place to ensure compliance.

Food safety systems need to keep pace with changes in climate, global food production, and supply systems that affect consumers, industry, and our planet.

Strategies for Sustainable Food: The Food System Approach

- *Increasing agriculture's low productivity* by addressing issues such as risks due to climate change, short-term weather anomalies, and natural resource degradation.
- *Promotion of healthy, low environmental impact diets* by framing policies to incentivize fruit and vegetable production and remove subsidies on less healthy foodstuffs, which also generally have higher greenhouse gas emissions, is required.
- *Diversification of diets* by increasing the variety of foods and food groups in the diet helps to ensure adequate intake of essential nutrients.
- *Food fortification* by the addition of nutrients, either by providing supplements such as vitamin A and iron pills/capsules (medical supplementation) or by adding micronutrients in food products.
- *Introducing biofortified varieties of crops* into the food chain to enable better health of human and animal populations.

Community Strategies to Clean Water

Water treatment before distribution is vital to ensure that only safe drinking water reaches households. Water sources also need protection from pesticide contamination and chemical contamination, and hence regulation of industrial effluents being released into water bodies and wastewater management are important.

World over, in all HICs and globally, making water safe or water purification at the source is known to be the best and most cost-effective method. Therefore, in all HICs, safe drinking water from the tap is a primary fundamental to life and dignity.

If 'at source' purification is not possible, then community-based strategies should be recommended. Every family having to make its water safe to drink is the most inefficient way forward. For communities/families, the method of purification recommended should be based on water quality. Filtration and chlorination are cost-effective methods. If reverse osmosis (RO) filtration is used, wastewater should be properly reused. For communities that rely on water sources at high risk of contamination with pathogens, the focus should be on household water treatment; safe storage of the treated water; and behavior change communication to improve hygiene, sanitation, and water-handling practices (https://www.cdc.gov/safewater/index.html). Water-saving devices should be fitted on taps and people should be encouraged to use water sparingly.

Emerging technologies on safe chemical-free sanitizers and disinfectants should be promoted.

Role of Regulatory Bodies in Achieving Food Safety

In India, the Food Safety and Standards Act 2006 is an integrated food law that consolidates all the laws relating to food safety or a single reference point for all matters relating to food safety and standards. It is primarily responsible for protecting and promoting public health through regulation and enforcement of food safety. Introducing the act has been a major paradigm shift from food safety in the marketplace to food safety along the supply chain from farm to table, ensuring that only safe foods are placed in the market.

India is also a cosignatory of the World Trade Organization and an active member of the Codex Alimentarius Commission, an international reference point for food trade that seeks food safety and consumer protection using scientific evidence. India has also proactively fostered partnerships with United Nations and its bodies such as the World Health Organization, Food and Agriculture Organization, and World Bank in achieving the 2030 Sustainable Development Goals.

However, despite having a robust legal framework in place, India still struggles with effectively enforcing food safety norms and standards. Standards are meaningless if there is no enforcement mechanism to ensure compliance.

CONCLUSION

Establishing a food safety culture in India would require coordinated action by a diverse group of stakeholders – the government at national, state, and local levels; food businesses; civil society and consumer organizations; food and nutrition professionals; farmers and farmers' organizations; science and research institutions; and others – using their combined skills, assets, and capabilities to achieve the shared goal.

A planetary health approach to the production of sustainable, nutritious, safe, and ethical food, delivered to all with minimal waste, will promote human, animal, and environmental well-being.

KEY MESSAGES

1. Unsafe food is a threat to human health and is responsible for foodborne illnesses globally. It contains microbiological, chemical, or physical hazards.
2. Effective food safety and quality control systems can safeguard the health and well-being of people.
3. Knowledge of food safety principles and food safety literacy is also important for ensuring safe food for all.
4. Having food safety ensured at a systems level, through stringent local, state, and country regulations and their implementation with diligent monitoring, evaluation, and accountability are critical to ensure safe food is available and accessible to all people.
5. Building food safety capacity and awareness among consumers is also important.
6. A planetary health approach to the production of sustainable, nutritious, safe, and ethical food, delivered to all with minimal waste, will promote human, animal, and environmental well-being.
7. There is no food security without food safety.

REFERENCES

Alders R. G., Ratanawongprasat N., Schönfeldt H., Stellmach D. A planetary health approach to secure, safe, sustainable food systems: Workshop report. *Food Security.* 2018 Apr; 10(2):489–93.

Arimond M., Wiesmann D., Becquey E. A., Carriquiry A., Daniels M., Deitchler M., Fanou N., Ferguson E., Joseph M., Kennedy G., Martin-Prével Y. *Dietary diversity as a measure of the micronutrient adequacy of women's diets in resource-poor areas: Summary of results from five sites.* Washington, DC: FANTA-2 Bridge, FHI. 2011; 360: 2011.

Community Water Centre, Clean Drinking Water Solution for Rural and Urban Communities, Booklet. (2021) WHO-UNICEF. Progress on household drinking water, sanitation and hygiene, 2000–2020: five years into the SDGs, Geneva: World Health Organization.

India Today. (2016). FSSAI to formulate new policies for food safety. Retrieved June 13, 2020, from *India Today.* http://indiatoday.intoday.in/story/fssai-to-formulate-new-policies-for-food-safety/1/599086.html

Marino, D. D. (2007). Water and food safety in the developing world: Global implications for health and nutrition of infants and young children. *J Am Diet Assoc.* 107:1930–1934

SEWAH. (2020). *Small water enterprises strategy to adapt during Covid-19.* SEWAH, Webinar Proceedings May 14, 2020.

Willett, W., Rockström J., Loken B., Springmann M., Lang T., Vermeulen S., Garnett T., Tilman D., DeClerck F., Wood A., Jonell M. (2019). Food in the Anthropocene: the EAT–Lancet Commission on healthy diets from sustainable food systems. *The Lancet.* Feb 2;393(10170):447–92.

WHO. (n.d.). *United Nations Interagency Task Force on the Prevention and Control of Non-Communicable Diseases: 2019–2021 strategy.* Geneva: WHO.

Yadava, D. K. (2018). Nutritional security through crop biofortification in India: Status & future prospects. *The Indian Journal of Medical Research.* 2018 Nov;148(5): 621

WEBSITES

UNIDO. 2015. Meeting Standards, Winning Markets – Trade Standards Compliance 2015. UNIDO/Norad/Institute of Development Studies, https://www.unido.org/our-focus/advancing-economic-competitiveness/meeting-standards/meeting-standards-winning-markets.

WHO International Food Safety Conference. 2019. The First FAO/WHO/AU International Food Safety Conference. https://www.who.int/docs/default-source/resources/chairpersons-summary-addis-ababa-en.pdf?sfvrsn=865efacf_6

Prüss-Ustün A., Wolf J., Bartram J., Clasen T., Cumming O., Freeman M.C., Gordon B., Hunter P. R., Medlicott K., Johnston R. Burden of disease from inadequate water, sanitation and hygiene for selected adverse health outcomes: An updated analysis with a focus on low- and middle-income countries. *Int J Hyg Environ Health.* 2019 Jun; 222(5): 765–777. doi: 10.1016/j.ijheh.2019.05.004. Epub 2019 May 12. PMID: 31088724; PMCID: PMC6593152.

https://www.who.int/foodsafety/areas_work/foodborne-diseases/ferg/en/

https://swachhbharatmission.gov.in/SBMCMS/about-us.htm#content

https://economictimes.indiatimes.com/news/economy/indicators/indias-gdp-grows-at-8-2-per-cent-in-2018-19

https://economictimes.indiatimes.com/news/economy/indicators/india-ranks-130-in-uns-human-development-index

https://www.un.org/sustainabledevelopment/sustainable-development-goals/

www.beyondcorona.in

www.ritewater.in

https://www.cdc.gov/safewater/index.html

https://ejalshakti.gov.in/JSA/JSA/Home.aspx

https://www.aquasana.com/info/education/boiled-water-vs-filtered-water

A Perspective: Evidence-based Cancer Control Interventions to Improve Population Health and Health Equity

Mark Parascandola

Substantial progress has been made in reducing cancer incidence and mortality through the introduction of evidence-based cancer prevention and control measures. However, the impact of these advances has not been distributed equitably throughout the globe. As the burden of cancer decreases among high-income countries (HICs), it continues to expand among low- and middle-income countries (LMICs), creating a growing disparity.[1]

As two chapters in this volume (Chapter 10 on cancer screening and Chapter 12 on health promotion) describe, there is a range of evidence-based cancer control interventions available at the individual, institutional, and policy levels. The U.S. National Cancer Institute's Evidence-Based Cancer Control Programs database, for example, includes over 200 entries.[2] Moreover, many cancers are preventable through reductions in risk factors (such as reducing tobacco and alcohol use, and vaccination against cancer-causing infections, including human papillomavirus and hepatitis B virus) and through screening and early detection.

However, a key challenge to reducing the global burden of cancer, particularly in LMICs, is the poor implementation of cancer prevention and control strategies that are known to work. For example, human papillomavirus vaccinations have been scaled up across many HICs, but implementation lags in LMICs. In response, the World Health Organization (WHO) launched a global initiative in 2020 that acknowledged the need to develop context-specific strategies to accelerate the elimination of cervical cancer across diverse settings.[3] The authors in this volume describe a range of challenges faced in implementing cancer control interventions in LMICs, ranging from lack of awareness among patients and practitioners to systemic challenges in delivering care where it is needed.

Greater attention is needed to understand the barriers to implementation and develop strategies to overcome them. Dissemination and implementation (D&I) science provides a set of principles, methods, and frameworks that promote the integration of evidence-based interventions and policies into real-world settings to improve population health and health equity.[4] The WHO has produced an Implementation Research Toolkit, and its global action plan for the prevention and control of noncommunicable diseases prioritized research agenda includes studying "contextual factors that affect research–policy–practice processes promoting the use of research findings."[5] Core D&I science concepts include an emphasis on stakeholder-driven agenda setting and collaborative problem-solving to relevance; a focus on analyzing multilevel contextual factors (e.g., political, organizational, and individual); the application of theoretical frameworks and implementation strategies; and an emphasis on measuring implementation outcome, including acceptability, feasibility, fidelity, adaptation, cost, sustainability, and equity.

Much of the current evidence for the implementation of cancer prevention and control interventions comes from HICs. However, intervention and implementation strategies developed in HICs may require adaptation for successful implementation in LMICs due to competing health priorities, resource limitations, health system structure, and social and cultural context.[6,7] The authors in this volume rightly emphasize the critical need for raising awareness and increasing health literacy about cancer to empower patients and communities and address stigma. Indeed, implementation of effective cancer control requires education and behavior change not only at the individual level but also at the system level. Advancing awareness of and capacity for implementation of effective cancer control in all settings is critical to reducing the global burden of cancer.

NOTES

1. Torre LA, Siegel RL, Ward EM, Jemal A. Global cancer incidence and mortality rates and trends – An update. *Cancer Epidemiol Biomarkers Prev.* 2016 Jan;25(1):16–27.

2. National Cancer Institute. Evidence-Based Cancer Control Programs database. Available at https://ebccp.cancercontrol.cancer.gov.

3. Das M. WHO launches strategy to accelerate elimination of cervical cancer. *Lancet Oncol.* 2021;22:20–21.

DOI: 10.1201/b23385-16

4. Brownson RC, Colditz GA, Proctor EK. *Dissemination and implementation research in health: Translating science to practice.* New York: Oxford University Press; 2017.

5. TDR Implementation Research Toolkit. Available at http://adphealth.org/irtoolkit/.

6. Mandal R, Basu P. Cancer screening and early diagnosis in low and middle income countries: Current situation and future perspectives. *Bundesgesundheitsblatt Gesundheitsforschung Gesundheitsschutz* 2018;61:1505–1512.

7. Shah SC, Kayamba V, Peek RM Jr, Heimburger D. Cancer control in low- and middle-income countries: Is it time to consider screening? *J Glob Oncol.* 2019;5:1–8.

10 Public Health Approaches in Cancer Screening and Prevention

Experiences from Ground Level

Sharmila A. Pimple and Gauravi A. Mishra

CONTENTS

> While implementing more strategic prevention, screening, and early detection efforts, we must not overlook important disparities in the receipt of evidence-based care that can reduce the burden of cancer in high-risk and vulnerable populations.
>
> **National Academy of Medicine, United States of America**

Considering the complexities involved in the delivery of cancer prevention and screening services in public health program settings, this chapter tries to identify barriers to the adoption and implementation of cancer screening services in developing countries like India. The barriers have been discussed under the following categories with relevant case studies: (1) barriers due to the lack of knowledge and awareness about cancer prevention, (2) public health system barriers, and (3) sociocultural barriers. Considering the wide diversity within India, in terms of socioeconomic conditions of the population and health system capabilities in different states including rural and urban differences, it is apt to formulate evidence-based strategies and approaches that are operationally feasible to address the issues that will benefit the majority of the population and health-delivery systems in the country. Adopting measures that will increase participation; maximize coverage; and offer good compliance to screening, diagnosis, and cancer treatment would help develop sustainable cancer prevention and screening program.

Noncommunicable diseases (NCDs) contribute to the majority of mortalities globally, and cancer is emerging as the leading cause of death [1]. Cancer incidence and mortality are rapidly growing worldwide with an estimated 18.1 million new cancer cases and 9.6 million cancer deaths in 2018. However, the most common cancers and the leading cause of cancer-related mortality vary substantially across different regions and countries mainly reflected by its socioeconomic development.

India is passing through an epidemiological and demographic transition leading to the emergence of NCDs as a major public health problem. The estimates of the burden of disease due to cancer have been made based on data from population-based cancer registries of the Indian Council of Medical Research (ICMR). According to GLOBOCAN 2018 data, there were 1,157,294 new cancer cases in India in both men and women, 784,821 deaths, and 22,58,208 people living with cancer (within 5 years of diagnosis) in 2018. The top five cancers that affect the Indian population are breast, oral, cervical, gastric, and lung [1, 2].

CANCER CONTROL IN INDIA

Over one-third of cancers are known to be preventable, and another one-third are potentially curable provided they are diagnosed at an early stage of the disease. The three most common cancers – oral, breast, and cervical – which contribute 60% of the total burden of cancers in the country, are most amenable to prevention, screening, and early detection. Yet, more than 70% of all cancers

DOI: 10.1201/b23385-17

in India are found when the disease is so advanced that treatment is much less effective. Also, the late stage of presentation does not seem to have changed much over the past 30 years. This may be due to the low priority given to NCDs and the absence of an adequate health infrastructure and trained manpower [2–4]. A similar pattern and state of healthcare development is observed in other developing countries within the region. Breast, lung, cervix uteri, lip and oral cavity, and colorectum cancers have emerged as the top five common cancers in both sexes in the World Health Organization's South-East Asia region (SEARO). Cancers of the lip and oral cavity are also the leading cause of cancer death among men in Sri Lanka and Bangladesh [1, 2]. This underscores the need for health promotion to be able to enable individuals to avail of services and demand an adequate and appropriate healthcare infrastructure.

Thus the task of implementing effective prevention and screening programs to control the preventable cancer burden in India and other developing country settings should not be underestimated. One of the effective ways to reduce our nation's burden from cancer is to ensure that good quality, organized, population-based screening services are available and accessible to the people. Sufficient evidence has been gathered over the last two decades about the relevance and effectiveness of low-cost technologies for the prevention and early detection of common cancers such as cervical, breast, and oral cancers that can be adopted even in low-resource settings with constraints on logistic, financial, health infrastructure, and trained manpower resources and helps find these diseases early when they are easiest to treat.

CANCER CONTROL AND SCREENING IN PUBLIC HEALTH SETTINGS

India had a National Cancer Control Programme that was established in 1975–1976. This has contributed to the development of regional cancer centers, oncology wings in medical colleges, and support for the purchase of teletherapy machines. However, the National Cancer Control Programme somehow lacked the required thrust for community-based strategies in the prevention and control of cancer. There has been an excessive reliance on treatment-oriented approaches, neglecting prevention strategies. In the years 2015 and 2016, India's National Institute of Health and Family Welfare (NIHFW) developed screening and management guidelines through an opportunistic screening approach for NCDs including that of common cancers that were initiated through the National Programme for the Prevention and Control of Cancer, Diabetes, Cardiovascular Diseases and Stroke (NPCDCS). These guidelines are currently focused on screening using visual inspection-based approaches to cervical cancer screening, namely, visual inspection with 4% acetic acid (VIA), clinical breast examination for breast cancer screening, and oral visual inspection for oral cancer screening within the current public health systems framework [5, 6].

However, despite the recommendations for population-based cancer screening services, the screening services are largely provided as opportunistic interventions, mostly at tertiary or secondary care facilities. Diagnostic infrastructure in the country is also limited especially in rural settings; most pathology/cytology and treatment facilities remain concentrated in urban areas of the country. Appropriate and effective linkages between primary care and secondary or tertiary care facilities for diagnosis and treatment are lacking or are nonexistent in places. From the general population's perspective, appropriate information, sensitization, awareness, and empowerment that facilitates healthcare navigation and thereby utilization of the existing services at the nearest point of contact with the primary healthcare system also need to be developed.

Along with the aforementioned infrastructure and logistic issues, cancer screening programs in India also pose formidable barriers to program implementation and adoption along with unique challenges of access to screening facilities, issues related to women's participation, referrals for positive screening, linkages to diagnosis, treatment, and repeat visits. These barriers, if not addressed at the population program level, may undermine the efforts for effective implementation of cervix cancer screening. Evidence-based strategies and approaches that are operationally feasible and that will increase participation, maximize coverage, and offer good compliance to screening, diagnosis, and precancer treatment would help develop sustainable programs. Considering the complexities involved in the delivery of screening services in public health programs and the diversity in India in terms of socioeconomic conditions of the population and health system capabilities in different states including rural and urban areas, it is apt to formulate a set of evidence-based recommendations that would benefit the majority of the population and health-delivery systems and may help adopt best practices in a wide range of situations stratified by resources for a sustainable program.

CURRENT BARRIERS TO CANCER PREVENTION AND SCREENING

Under the World Health Organization's universal health coverage (UHC) and the health-related Sustainable Development Goal (SDG) targets for South-East Asia, there were substantial improvements in service coverage, with a regional average of 61% in 2019 compared with 46% in 2010. Many member states are introducing screening programs for selected preventable cancers such as cervical, breast, and oral. Population-level implementation of screening programs is at different stages of introduction in the region. Countries such as Bhutan, the Democratic People's Republic of Korea, and Thailand have reported more than 50% coverage for cervical cancer screening programs. However, coverage remains abysmally low in most other member countries in the region. Sri Lanka remains a case in point with targeted measures that were adopted to improve screening rates to 23%.

Although significant progress has been made in developing necessary operational guidelines for implementation in public health program settings, screening rates for oral, breast, and cervical cancers have not improved and are unacceptably low in India.

Some of the commonly identified barriers to the uptake of cancer screening services in developing countries generally can be categorized into (1) barriers due to lack of knowledge and awareness about cancer, (2) public health systems barriers, and (3) sociocultural barriers and women-specific personal barriers.

Cancer Literacy for Cancer Prevention and Screening

Barriers Due to Perceptions

Perception-related barriers include a lack of awareness and information about risk factors and the development of preventable common cancers, the need to screen the disease when healthy, where and how to access screening services if available, the screening process, and the benefits of early detection and treatment. The notion of seeking health services only upon having symptoms is largely prevalent. Many do not perceive the possibility of developing cancers and hence do not consider themselves candidates for screening [7–9].

Overall anxiety and fear of undertaking the screening test, how the test is going to be administered, perceived association with pain and discomfort, and the possibility of a positive result have been the main factors preventing the eligible population from participating in screening programs [10, 11].

Multiple studies have investigated the association of health literacy in molding cancer-related attitudes and behaviors to understand decision-making and improved health-seeking behavior [12–15]. A systematic review of the literature on health literacy has demonstrated the association of lower health literacy with poorer health behaviors and adverse health outcomes [16–18]. Health literacy is significantly intertwined with socioeconomic status.

Awareness about cancer risk factors, prevention, and currently available modalities for screening and early detection needs to be disseminated across all levels and sections of society to mobilize communities for the need and acceptance of such services. The first step toward achieving the goal for cancer education for populations is the development of appropriate, optimal information and education materials, and devising communication strategies that help populations to make informed decisions about participating in cancer screening programs.

We advocate the integration of the following important principles and guidelines for cancer literacy in delivering cancer education to address the barriers for communities not participating in cancer screening programs.

Essential Components of Cancer Awareness Education Program

A cancer education program should be formulated by incorporating some basic principles to optimize the content, messaging, and delivery of the same for meaningful impact to translate information into action for program participation.

1. The education content. The basic information should impart knowledge about common risk factors leading to cancers, specific symptoms and signs to identify them, the need to approach the nearest health facility, and the current available simple testing modalities to detect them as per the recommendations of the national guidelines. The importance of screening for the disease, the availability of treatment, and the possibility of a cure if detected early should be shared. Explaining the simplicity of performing the tests and ease of administering the primary cancer screening tests is equally important for program participation.

2. Communicating health information using plain language and simple terms that lend clarity for common people to understand and assimilate information is a very essential aspect of cancer education.
3. Addressing the common myths, misconceptions, and community perceptions about cancer and cancer screening is crucial for allaying anxiety and fears about participating in screening programs.
4. Text in local vernacular language with pictorial depiction facilitates conveying the messages more effectively.
5. The core messages about the overall benefits of participating in a cancer screening program, and that adopting risk prevention behavior and necessary modifications in lifestyle and participating in cancer screening can save lives need to be stressed during awareness-building.
6. Gender-neutral cancer education programs. Cancer awareness programs involving male family members are known to improve acceptance of screening programs, but at the same time may embarrass women when discussing their health-related issues in an open forum. Consensus and comfort of the target women audience involving direct face-to-face cancer education programs are important before considering gender-neutral cancer education programs. The involvement of local groups, such as teachers, local leaders, and religious leaders, impacts building trust and endorsement for the screening program.
7. Platforms for cancer awareness and education. Community outreach initiatives seeking the target audiences in their local communities are the best way to impart the information. A locally organized group education program is more likely to be well attended, facilitating more interaction. However, the target audience should be accessed at all opportunities including waiting areas and outpatient clinics for other health facilities such as other health and welfare activities.
8. Cancer education can be conducted by all levels of healthcare givers including trained health workers, midwives, nurses, and doctors.
9. Education tools. Depending on the resources available, imparting information with well-designed flip charts, calendar charts, slide shows, and video films including street plays can be organized. A government-channelized broad-based media campaign utilizing print and electronic media can improve the overall visibility of the program and enhance participation in screening programs.
10. Piloting the planned program interventions in representative communities and population groups to assess the local cultural acceptability of the desired intervention can help to tailor the interventions for that community and region. The pilot program might help predict the communication gaps and understanding of the messages to avoid spreading rumors and misinformation that can impact the entire implementation plan.

Public Health Program Barriers

Public Health Infrastructure

Efforts should be built on existing public health infrastructure and capacity to increase participation in cancer screening programs. The public health infrastructure needs to be equipped and scaled up to ensure sustainable and effective implementation of cancer screening programs to achieve the desired cancer prevention and screening goals. The majority of current cancer screening services are opportunistic in nature, offering cancer screenings to people when they visit health facilities for other medical reasons. The existing pattern of rendering opportunistic screening services needs to be modified to expand and organize the cancer screening program at the primary care level. However, infrastructure barriers along with a lack of trained manpower resources have been challenging to India's fragmented healthcare system for the widespread implementation of organized screening programs. Ease of availability, access to the health system, cost of services, and perceived quality of services are some of the determinants for participation in screening programs.

Quality of Services and Attitudes of Health Personnel

Government rollout of cancer screening activities endorses the need for the program, but participation in the program is mainly driven by the ease of access to the services, and conditions of the health facilities determine women's satisfaction with the services they receive. The negative attitudes of health care personnel, especially nurses and other paramedical workers, toward women were mentioned as an important factor in the utilization of cancer screening services [19].

The rapport and trust with the health staff influence participation. A negative experience in the form of unfriendly surroundings and staff will impact the uptake of services. Since women's screening for breast and cervical cancer involves examination of the private parts, the nature of privacy accorded to the participating women, pain, discomfort during the examination, and the indifferent attitude of the health staff during examination also determines how communities participate in the program. All the above also negatively impacts other community members participating in the screening activities [19, 20].

Social and Cultural Barriers as Determinants of Participation

Social determinants of health are vital for overall public health achievement. Social and cultural perceptions can discourage eligible individuals, especially women, from seeking screening services.

The majority of the women who attend and access opportunistic screening services are often screened on the recommendation and referral of their local health provider since they are experiencing certain symptoms [21, 22]. The general population is not aware of the need to undergo screening tests to detect diseases when they are apparently normal. The fundamental knowledge and benefits of screening are nonexistent. Efforts are needed to increase the target population's knowledge and awareness of common cancers, especially the screening methods, and to improve their perceptions of the screening process. Evidence from Asia, Africa, and Latin America suggests that many women do not know about cervical and breast cancer screening, and are not aware of what types of services are available or where and when to seek them [21–32].

In the context of cervical cancer screening, knowledge about human papillomavirus (HPV) as a sexually transmitted infection can lead to communities stigmatizing screening, causing embarrassment for women who present for screening services. For women, the healthcare provider for screening should be female, as the presence of male health providers can adversely impact screening participation [21, 22, 25–31]. Women's participation in the screening program is also decided by the combined decision of extended family members (mother-in-law) and husband who need to be made knowledgeable about the benefits of the screening program.

The fear and anxiety of being diagnosed with cancer and thereby attracting social stigma for herself and the family weighs equally heavy on the minds of women, especially in communities where families bear the brunt of social stigma due to cancer.

The travel time to access services, ease of availability of transportation, loss of wages, and the competing priorities of child care and routine family chores impact the motivation and decision to participate in the screening program. Lack of sufficient privacy, cultural modesty, embarrassment to disrobe for the pelvic examination necessary for cervical cancer screening, and concerns about being attended to by or observed in the presence of male healthcare providers are important determinants for program participation by women [32].

CONCLUSIONS

Studies across multiple low- and middle-resource settings stress the importance of cancer literacy with appropriate information and communications channels to provide needed information about the benefits of cancer screenings. The sensitization of the target populations can generate community support and help inform decision-making for program participation. Communication channels should adopt cancer education messages that reduce fear, misconceptions, and stigma, and mobilize communities to accept cancer screening services [32].

From the public health program perspective, adequate training, and capacity building of the healthcare providers in administering quality cancer screening services that are accessible, easy to travel to, and of low cost are critical to increasing community participation in cancer screening programs [33]. Further mechanisms to track suspect positive cases that need follow-up must be developed. The referral pathways for further diagnosis and treatment need to be identified and further strengthened to facilitate and enable individuals with a positive screening test to access the diagnostic services, to return for possible treatment, and to return to the clinic for follow-up evaluation, which is an important component to the success of a screening program. The nearest accessible first-referral level unit needs to be identified and equipped to provide the needed care and at the same time avoid overburdening tertiary care systems. Adherence to the referral system guidelines and accountability at each level will help improvement in existing referral systems in

India. Patient navigation has come across as an important element that can facilitate improved healthcare access to overcome healthcare system barriers and facilitate timely access to medical facilities from screening to diagnosis to all phases of the cancer care continuum. Trained community health workers and village volunteers can be valuable patient navigators and resources to decrease the numbers lost to follow-up and thereby impact the efficiency of screening programs [48, 49].

BOX 10.1 CANCER LITERACY: CANCER EDUCATION MESSAGING

Building on the research evidence of the effectiveness of simple, low-cost technologies for early detection of common cancers of the cervix, breast, and oral cavity, Tata Memorial Centre, a recognized comprehensive cancer care center in Mumbai, India, developed a Rural Model District Cancer Control Programme that was initiated in 2003 as part of the tenth five-year plan project under the Department of Atomic Energy, Government of India. The population-based cancer screening program was implemented in two rural districts of Maharashtra State in Western India. No screening program is possible without adequate community awareness about preventable cancers. The aim of raising awareness is to make sure that a high proportion of the target population participates in the program. Women and men from every household in respective village campaigns were sought by the team of health workers and social workers to participate in cancer awareness programs or were given specific health messages to encourage them to participate in screening services. Implementation of community cancer awareness programs, however, underwent a lot of changes and transitions in the context of providing correct, relevant, and essential information related to the prevention, screening, and management of common cancers. Community cancer awareness programs conducted for various categories across the social ladder formed the platform and foundation on which relied the success of the rest of the program. The various stakeholders from the community were contacted for common cancer awareness and sensitization about the need for cancer screening services for the region, which included not only the population groups at the village level but targeted special focus groups such as the women's groups, local political leaders, school teachers, village-level primary healthcare workers, and local physicians and practitioners of alternative medicines. Awareness about preventable cancers and early detection tools was highly lacking not only across all segments of the population but among the practitioners of medicine as well. Thus, cancer awareness sessions in the population subgroups remain the backbone of the cancer screening services in the region [11, 18].

Cancer awareness program strategies involved reaching men and women with the same health awareness messages about the importance of oral, breast, and cervical cancer prevention to make them understand their role as motivators of women in the family and to support their partners to be screened and treated. In the Indian cultural context where men are decision-makers about important health issues concerning women in the family, the success of screening for breast or cervical cancer might depend on how effectively men can be educated about the benefits of these interventions. Reaching men within the community in a conservative culture with the same health awareness messages about the importance of breast and cervical cancer prevention was a daunting task, but did make a good impact in motivating their partners to be screened and treated when necessary [11, 18].

BOX 10.2 CANCER LITERACY: ADVERSE IMPACT OF FACTUAL INFORMATION SHARING FOR CANCER EDUCATION AND LESSONS LEARNED

Some of the information shared during cancer awareness and education sessions is about the risk factors for cervical cancers, which includes infection by HPV that can lead to development of cervical cancers. Risk factor information further includes which women are likely to get cervical cancers, which mentions HPV as a sexually transmitted disease (STD). Women with multiple sexual partners, sexual promiscuity by either partner, and bad genital hygiene could be the risk factors for the development of the disease. STDs are closely associated with stigma. People who have STDs are often stigmatized as once practicing excessive sexual activities or sexual immorality [34, 35].

In the Indian social-cultural context, due to the linkage of cervical cancer to risk factors such as HPV infection, which is acquired through sexual contact, particularly by those with a promiscuous sex life, the disease remains taboo, leading to women trying to delineate and disassociate themselves from having such risk factors. The stigma associated with STDs acted as a potential barrier for women to participate in cervical screening programs [36, 37].

In our experience, when women community leaders were contacted for understanding reasons for poor participation in cancer screening program the response was, "Our community women do not belong to the category of risk factors mentioned in your cancer education program. Our women come from respected families and practice very moral behavior. Women are embarrassed to participate and also fear being looked upon suspiciously by other community female members for immoral behavior". Similar feedback and responses were received from other communities too, which prompted us to restructure the content of the cervical cancer education program by avoiding the reference to sexually transmitted infection and laying more emphasis on the benefits of screening rather than risk factors. This experience in implementing strategies for participation in cancer screening programs brought out the fact that lack of awareness and stigma attached to STDs can function as a great barrier to health promotion, diagnosis, and treatment, and should be accompanied by extensive health education to inform women and to destigmatize HPV infection.

BOX 10.3 CANCER LITERACY: AVOIDING RUMORS AND MISINFORMATION

Cancer education messages need to impart appropriate information about the screening procedure and the process for undertaking a cancer screening test. If individuals are informed about what to expect from a procedure, it helps lends clarity and develop trust in the system. Gaps in understanding of the exact nature of the screening process can lead to misinformation and also rumors and suspicion about the screening procedures.

One of the major rumors and misinformation that was largely believed by some of the women that prevented many communities from participating was that the screening process involves removal of the uterus or some other organs as part of the organ transfer racket and also that they might contract other diseases such as HIV. Awareness and explanation about the screening procedure during cancer education sessions and also as part of the pretest counseling session are extremely important to avoid the spread of such misinformation.

BOX 10.4 PUBLIC HEALTH PROGRAM BARRIERS: COMMUNICATION AND NETWORKING WITH LOCAL COMMUNITIES AND STAKEHOLDERS

Organizing community cancer screening services in the adopted rural and urban areas was an uphill task, especially in conservative rural communities with illiteracy, ignorance, prevalent caste culture, local politics, and suspicious attitudes toward the screening services. Women in poor urban and rural communities were unaware of any cancer risks nor options for and access to cancer screenings. It was possible to overcome these hurdles by selecting and identifying local volunteers, political, and religious leaders to initially educate and sensitize them about the benefits of the cancer screening program before taking up cancer literacy and awareness programs for the larger communities and population. Sensitizing the local leaders and stakeholders helped create a strong sense of community ownership of the program along with building trust in the community by seeing their local leaders talking positively about the need and benefits of participating in such programs. Also, healthcare staff from the public health program was trained in delivering cancer education and communication skills, and good community networking with key local leaders/women's groups and other welfare groups thus enabling them to get consistently good community participation in screening activities.

BOX 10.5 PUBLIC HEALTH PROGRAM BARRIERS: DIFFICULTIES IN ACCESSING AND NAVIGATING THE HEALTHCARE SYSTEM

Issues related to access to the health system such as no knowledge of the health system and how to use it, geographic location, proximity to facility and availability of transportation facilities, time taken to travel to the facility, and culture. Difficulty in navigating healthcare facilities and services was reported as one of the prominent barriers to accessing screening as well as further diagnosis and treatment facilities post-screening. Lack of adequate information about the exact location, transportation to the facility, where and when to obtain the required service, multiple examination requirements, ability to meet or access the specialty or expert on the same day, uncertainty of the availability of the required service on the same day, and repeated visits have been seen as a major deterrent individuals face from accessing available services [38]. Long wait times for screenings in the hospital leading to disruption of work, and neglect of family and children, especially among nursing mothers, were identified as barriers to cancer screening programs especially when they do not have apparent disease systems [39].

BOX 10.6 PUBLIC HEALTH PROGRAM BARRIERS: LACK OF TRUST IN THE HEALTHCARE DELIVERY SYSTEM

Low levels of trust in the healthcare system along with bad previous experiences with the health system and health professionals are important factors for program participation. When invited to participate in the screening program, some of the participants expressed a lack of confidence in the healthcare system concerning the quality of the services, the safety of the procedures undertaken, perceived harm arising from undergoing screening examinations such as using the same instruments without sterilization, and fear of being infected with other diseases either from the screening equipment or from other sources or procedures within the healthcare facility. Along with fears of an adverse finding, there was concern about the disclosure of a positive screening result and fear of dissemination of the information in neighboring communities with consequential social isolation.

BOX 10.7 PUBLIC HEALTH PROGRAM BARRIERS: NEED FOR SINGLE-VISIT APPROACHES FOR SCREENING AND TREATMENT TO PREVENT DROP OUT

Women with abnormal test results or positive results on primary screening at the primary care level require attendance at secondary or tertiary healthcare facilities for confirmation of diagnosis and further treatment if required. This requires a functional and effective referral system as well as well-equipped and trained personnel to undertake diagnostic confirmation and requisite treatment. However, many of the public health facilities in secondary and tertiary care settings are lacking due to the paucity or nonavailability of specialized and trained medical staff, which can give rise to long waiting hours and repeat visits due to the nonavailability of equipment and health personnel. This is likely to impact the uptake of services by patients being unwilling to return for another visit, reluctant to follow-up for diagnosis or return for future screenings [23, 24].

The evidence-based recommended test of VIA for low-resource settings gives immediate results, which when linked to cryotherapy facilities permit a single-visit screen and treatment strategy. The World Health Organization has recommended VIA-based screen-and-treat programs for better compliance with cervical precancer treatment, especially in regions with poor access to healthcare facilities [40–42]. Cryotherapy-based treatment in single-visit approaches, when conducted by competent providers, has been shown to be safe, feasible, and acceptable with over 85% or greater cure rates [43].

BOX 10.8 SOCIAL AND CULTURAL BARRIERS: STIGMA OF CANCER AS CONTAGIOUS

In our program implementation, after participating in a cancer screening program, some women preferred privacy and confidentiality of communicating a positive screening report to only themselves and not to their accompanying women friends or close relatives including husbands. Women anticipated discrimination stemming from the belief of cancer is contagious. There was fear of stigma associated with a diagnosis of cancer and being ostracized from the community and family. There were instances of refusals to referrals to higher health facilities and follow-up during house visits undertaken by medical social workers or health workers of screen-positive women for further diagnosis and treatment. Participants feared they would face severe forms of social discrimination from being labeled as cancer patients.

A public education program was then structured to include the misconceptions related to cancer diagnosis and to decrease stigma associated with cancer in terms of it being noncontagious; caring for cancer patients; and sharing space, food, and clothes. This was crucial in promoting prevention, early detection, and treatment of cancer. Perception and belief of a fatalistic outcome of a positive screening result are extensively reported in many studies as a barrier to uptaking screening [19, 20, 44].

BOX 10.9 SOCIAL AND CULTURAL STIGMATIZATION: DISCRIMINATION TOWARD DAUGHTERS IN FAMILIES WITH A CANCER MEMBER

Fearing a positive outcome of a screening test had another dimension of the discrimination of the family and victimization of the daughters of the family. In individual counseling of the suspect cases of women participants, it was revealed that the women did not want the disclosure of their suspect positive results in front of other community members or close family members. Certain sections of women feared their daughters would be discriminated against because the community links a mother's cancer to the future occurrence of the same with her daughters. Therefore, the daughters were thus targeted as noneligible for marriage out of the perceived notion and fear of transmitting the disease to their daughters: "like mother, like daughter," or likely to get cancer just like their mothers. The suspect mothers strongly discouraged house visits by healthcare workers for any kind of follow-up examination and treatment as these visits by healthcare staff were looked upon by the community as communication of an urgent and probably fatal outcome of the screening program. The counseling of the family and especially the daughters was undertaken in the demonstration program.

BOX 10.10 SOCIAL AND CULTURAL BARRIERS: BARRIERS TO ACCEPT TREATMENT IN THE ABSENCE OF VISIBLE SYMPTOMS

Screening is defined as the presumptive identification of unrecognized disease in an apparently healthy, asymptomatic population using tests and examinations. Cervical cancer screening involves testing for precancer and cancer among women who have no symptoms and may feel perfectly healthy. Cervical precancerous lesions, if detected during the screening program, can be easily treated, preventing the development and progression of invasive cervical cancer. The effectiveness of a screening program largely depends on linking screening to treatment. An important barrier faced by the cervical cancer screening programs was women accepting and participating in cervical precancer treatment once found positive on a screening test. The presence of cervical precancer lesions does not cause or give rise to any symptoms for the women. For the majority of Indian women, like in many parts of the world, visiting a physician are for reasons of illness or manifest symptoms and not for prevention.

The general population associates treatment with the manifestation of disease symptoms and since women detected with cervical precancer do not suffer from any symptoms, the program staff was facing difficulties counseling and convincing women to take treatment. Women did not perceive or feel the urgency to take further treatment for cervical precancer. Reasons quoted for noncompliance to accessing and seeking treatment included, "Family members do not think there is need to take treatment since I do not suffer from any symptoms" and "My family consulted our local doctor and since I do not have symptoms my family physician, local health practitioner suggested that I need not undergo any treatment", findings consistent with other studies in low- and middle-income settings [27, 45].

Other reasons for noncompliance to treatment were also attributed to distance to the hospital, the requirement of an accompanying person, anxiety about navigating the health system to the appropriate health facility, repeat visits due to the nonavailability of health staff, and competing family priorities, among others.

These reasons for noncompliance were supported by the findings of cancer screening studies in Mumbai and rural South India, which identified the opinion of the spouse, the local doctor's role, and family obligations as the main reasons for noncompliance [46, 47]. Incorporating and imparting a better understanding of the precancer disease stage and the importance of treatment needs appropriate counseling of the women and family members for improving spousal and family support for better implementation and success of the program.

REFERENCES

1. Ferlay J, Colombet M, Soerjomataram I, Mathers C, Parkin DM, Piñeros M, Znaor A, Bray F. Estimating the global cancer incidence and mortality in 2018: GLOBOCAN sources and methods. *Int J Cancer.* 2018 Oct 23. https://doi.org/10.1002/ijc.31937.

2. Bray F, Ferlay J, Soerjomataram I, Siegel RL, Torre LA, Jemal A. Global cancer statistics 2018: GLOBOCAN estimates of incidence and mortality worldwide for 36 cancers in 185 countries. *CA Cancer J Clin.* 2018 Nov;68(6):394–424.

3. Torre LA, Bray F, Siegel RL, Ferlay J, Lortet-Tieulent J, Jemal A. Global cancer statistics, 2012. *CA: Cancer J Clin.* 2015;65:87–108.

4. Fitzmaurice C, Dicker D, Pain A, et al. The global burden of cancer 2013. *Global Burden of Disease Cancer Collaboration: JAMA Oncology.* 2015;1:505–527.

5. *Operational Guidelines for Common Non–Communicable Diseases. Report of the Task Force on Comprehensive Primary Health Care Rollout.* Ministry of Health and Family Welfare, Government of India, 2015. Available from: http://www.nicpr.res.in/images/pdf/guidelines_for_population_level_screening_of_common_NCDs.pdf

6. *Operational Framework: Management of Common Cancers.* Ministry of Health and Family Welfare Government of India. Available from: http://cancerindia.org.in/wp- content/uploads/2017/11/Operational_Framework_Management_of_Common_Cancers.pdf

7. Gu C, Chan CW, Twinn S. How sexual history and knowledge of cervical cancer and screening influence Chinese women's screening behavior in mainland China. *Cancer Nurs* 2010;33:445–453.

8. Fylan F Screening for cervical cancer: A review of women's attitudes, knowledge, and behaviour. *Br J Gen Pract* 1998;48:1509–1514.

9. Ackerson K, Preston SD. A decision theory perspective on why women do or do not decide to have cancer screening: Systematic review. *J Adv Nurs* 2009;65:1130–1140.

10. Das BC, Hussain S, Nasare V, Bharadwaj M. Prospects and prejudices of human papillomavirus vaccines in India vaccine. *Vaccine* 2008;26:2669–2679.

11. Shastri S, Pimple S, Mishra G, Patil S, Banvali S. Indian communities participating in controlling women's cancers. *Health in South: East Asia, SEARO Newsletter.* World Health Organization. September Edition 5(2). ISSN 2070-6804.

12. Davis TC, Williams MV, Marin E, Parker RM, Glass J. Health literacy and cancer communication. *CA Cancer J Clin.* 2002;52(3):134–149.

13. Morris NS, Field TS, Wagner JL, Cutrona SL, Roblin DW. The association between health literacy and cancer-related attitudes, behaviors, and knowledge. *J Health Commun.* 2013;18(suppl 1):233–241. https://doi.org/10.1080/10810730.2013.825667.

14. Mazor KM, Rubin DL, Roblin DW, et al. Health literacy-listening skill and patient questions following cancer prevention and screening discussions. *Health Expect.* 2015;19(4):920–934. https://doi.org/ 10.1111/hex.12387.

15. Ownby RL, Acevao A, Waldrop-Valverde D, Jacobs RJ, Caballero J. Abilities, skills and knowledge in measures of health literacy. *Patient Educ Couns.* 2014;95(2):211–217. https://doi.org/10.1016/j.pec.2014.02.002.

16. Oldach BR, Katz ML. Health literacy and cancer screening: A systematic review. *Patient Educ Couns.* 2014 February;94(2):149–157.

17. Berkman ND, Sheridan SL, Donahue KE, Halpern DJ, Viera A, Crotty K, Holland A, Brasure M, Lohr KN, Harden E, Tant E, Wallace I, Viswanathan M. Health literacy interventions and outcomes: An updated systematic review. *Evid Rep Technol Assess.* March 2011;199:1–941.

18. Dinshaw KA, Shastri SS, Patil SS. Community intervention for cancer control & prevention: Lessons learnt. *Indian J Pediat Med Oncol.* 2004;25:4–8.

19. Lim JNW, Ojo AA. Barriers to utilisation of cervical cancer screening in Sub Sahara Africa: A systematic review. *Eur J Cancer Care.* 2017;26:e12444. https://doi.org/10.1111/ecc.12444

20. Azami-Aghdash S, Ghojazadeh M, Sheyklo SG, Daemi A, Kolahdouzan K, Mohseni M, Moosavi A. Breast cancer screening barriers from the woman's perspective: A meta-synthesis. *Asian Pac J Cancer Prev.* 2015; 16(8):3463–3471.

21. Leyva M, Byrd T, Tarwater P. Attitudes towards cervical cancer screening: A study of beliefs among women in Mexico. *Californian J Health Promotion.* 2006;4(2):13–24.

22. Ncube B, Bey A, Knight J, et al. Factors associated with the uptake of cervical cancer screening among women in Portland, Jamaica. *North Am J Med Sci.* 2015;7(3):104–113.

23. Tripathi N, Kadam YR, Dhobale RV, Gore AD. Barriers for early detection of cancer amongst Indian rural women. *South Asian J Cancer.* 2014 Apr;3(2):122–7.

24. Kadam YR, Quraishi SR, Dhoble RV, Sawant MR, Gore AD. Barriers for early detection of cancer amongst urban Indian women: A cross sectional study. *Iran J Cancer Prev.* 2016 Feb; 9(1):e3900. Epub 2016 Feb 22.

25. Winkler J, Bingham A, Coffey P, et al. Women's participation in a cervical cancer screening program in northern Peru. *Health Educ. Res.* 2008;23(1):10–24.

26. Fort VK, Makin MS, Siegler AJ, et al. Barriers to cervical cancer screening in Mulanje, Malawi: A qualitative study. *Patient Pref Adherence* 2011;5:125–131.

27. Ansink AC, Tolhurst R, Haque R, et al. Cervical cancer in Bangladesh: Community perceptions on cervical cancer and cervical cancer screening. *Trans R Soc Trop Med Hygiene* 2008;102(5):499–505.

28. Mupepi SC, Sampselle CM, Johnson TRB. Knowledge, attitudes, and demographic factors influencing cervical cancer screening behavior of Zimbabwean women. *Journal of Women's Health* 2011;20(6):943–952.

29. Ndikom CM, Ofi BA. Awareness, perception and factors affecting utilization of cervical cancer screening services among women in Ibadan, Nigeria: A qualitative study. *Reproductive Health* 2012;9:11.

30. Wong LP, Wong YL, Low WY, et al. Knowledge and awareness of cervical cancer and screening among Malaysian women who have never had a Pap smear: A qualitative study. *Singapore Med J*. 2009;50(1):49–53.

31. Modibbo FI, Dareng E, Bamisaye P, et al. Qualitative study of barriers to cervical cancer screening among Nigerian women. *BMJ Open* 2016;6:e008533.

32. Sievers D and White H. *Evidence Series: Cervical Cancer Screening and Prevention, and Barriers to Uptake*. Washington, DC: Population Services International; 2016.

33. Lu, M., Mortiz S., Lorenzetti D., et al. A systematic review of interventions to increase breast and cervical cancer screening uptake among Asian women. *BMC Public Health* 2012;12:413.

34. Smith RA, Ferrara M, Witte K. Social sides of health risks: Stigma and collective efficacy. *Health Commun*. 2007;21(1):55–64.

35. Lichtenstein B, Hook EW, Sharma AK. Public tolerance, private pain: Stigma and sexually transmitted infections in the American Deep South. *Cult Health Sex*. 2005 Jan;7(1):43–57.

36. Cunningham SD, Tschann J, Gurvey JE, Fortenberry JD, Ellen JM. Attitudes about sexual disclosure and perceptions of stigma and shame. *Sex Transm Infect*. 2002 Oct; 78(5):334–8.

37. Fortenberry JD, McFarlane M, Bleakley A, Bull S, Fishbein M, Grimley DM, et al. Relationships of stigma and shame to gonorrhea and HIV screening. *Am J Public Health*. 2002;92(3):378–381. https://doi.org/10.2105/AJPH.92.3.378

38. Fort VK, Makin MS, Siegler AJ, Ault K, Rochat R. Barriers to cervical cancer screening in Mulanje, Malawi: A qualitative study. *Patient Pref Adherence* 2011;5:125–131.

39. Ngugi CW, Boga H, Muigai AWT, Wanzala P, Mbithi J. Factors affecting uptake of cervical cancer early detection measures among women in Thika, Kenya. *Health Care for Women International* 2012;33:595–613.

40. Sankaranarayanan R, Rajkumar R, Esmy PO, et al. Effectiveness, safety and acceptability of 'see and treat' with cryotherapy by nurses in a cervical screening study in India. *Br J Cancer*. 2007;96:738–743.

41. Sherris J, Wittet S, Kleine A, et al. Evidence-based, alternative cervical cancer screening approaches in low resource settings. *Int Perspect Sexual Reprod Health*. 2009;35:147–154.

42. Denny L, Kuhn L, De Souza M, Pollack AE, Dupree W, Wright TC. Screen-and-treat approaches for cervical cancer prevention in low-resource settings: A randomized controlled trial. *JAMA*. 2005;294:2173–2181.

43. Castro W, Gage J, Gaffikin L, et al. *Effectiveness, Safety and Acceptability of Cryotherapy: A Systematic Literature Review.* Seattle: PATH; 2003. Cervical Cancer Prevention Issues in Depth, No. 1.

44. Williams M, Kuffour G, Ekuadzi E, Yeboah M, ElDuah M and Tuffour P. Assessment of psychological barriers to cervical cancer screening among women in Kumasi, Ghana using a mixed methods approach. *African Health Sci.* 2013;13:1054–1060.

45. Lyimo FS, Beran TN. Demographic, knowledge, attitudinal, and accessibility factors associated with uptake of cervical cancer screening among women in a rural district of Tanzania: Three public policy implications. *BMC Public Health* 2012;12:22.

46. Dinshaw K, Mishra G, Shastri S, Badwe R, Kerkar R, Ramani S, Thakur M, Uplap P, Kakade A, Gupta S, Ganesh B. Determinants of compliance in a cluster randomised controlled trial on screening of breast and cervix cancer in Mumbai, India: Compliance to referral and treatment. *Oncology* 2007;73:154–161.

47. Sankaranarayanan R, Rajkumar R, Arrossi S, Theresa R, Esmy PO, Mahé C, Muwonge R, Parkin DM, Cherian J. Determinants of participation of women in a cervical cancer visual screening trial in rural south India. *Cancer Detect Prev.* 2003; 27(6):457–65.

Case Study: *Application of Health Promotion for Cancer Prevention: Lessons from the Field*

Suma Nair, Thejas Kathrikolly and Jayasree Ramachandran

CONTENTS

BACKGROUND

The decadal shift from communicable to noncommunicable diseases and a resultant increase in cancer burden in low- and middle-income countries has been compellingly illustrated by the global burden of disease data.[1] India is no exception to this increasing burden and reports over 11 lakh new cases and 7 lakh deaths annually.[2] Although the exact disease burden is difficult to capture due to the nonuniform coverage of existing and limited population-based cancer registries, available data indicate not only a high age-adjusted incidence rate but also a high mortality-to-incidence ratio for certain cancers.[3,4] Studies have pointed toward a delayed diagnosis, leading to ineffective treatment and a reduced survival rate.[5,6] Low awareness about the disease coupled with poor accessibility and affordability appears to be the three most important factors responsible for this bleak situation.[7] Health promotion, with its tenets of creating a supportive environment for improving health and reducing health inequalities, was considered the best approach in this setting to bring about a desirable change in cancer prevention and control.

CENTRE FOR COMMUNITY ONCOLOGY: A CANCER PREVENTION INITIATIVE IN COASTAL KARNATAKA

This initiative was commenced with the objective of implementing primary, secondary, and tertiary levels of prevention with respect to common cancers in the region.

We pilot-tested a primary prevention strategy in the field practice area of community medicine, comprised of 50,000 people spread across 11 villages. Although the area boasts a commendable female literacy rate and favorable sex ratio, health literacy and particularly cancer literacy were poor.[8] This also translated into the delayed presentation of cancer cases with a significant impact on the five-year survival rate.[9]

Subsequent to the test run, the following strategies were adopted to scale up the health promotion activities across the district:

1. Community profiling using qualitative study methods

   Focus group discussions (FGDs) among community participants helped us to map their needs and barriers and enabled the development of customized messages and targeted methods.

2. Engaging a designated patient advocate

   A remarkable finding from the FGDs was the unanimous request for a liaising person between the community and the tertiary care hospital. The participants felt this would enhance uptake and improve accessibility as people especially from rural settings are intimidated by the tertiary or secondary care hospital surroundings. This led us to engage a patient advocate who not only sets up awareness camps but also liaises with the participants throughout the cancer care continuum.

3. Enhancing community engagements

   Being accepted by the community is crucial to the success of a community-based health promotion initiative. Effective engagement with the community can be achieved by collaborating with influential community and nongovernmental organizations. In addition, apprising government leaders and volunteering to partner with them is a win-win situation for the community at large. This not only results in delivering quality healthcare service for the larger

 DOI: 10.1201/b23385-18

expanse of the population but also knowledge sharing for better care. Another valuable addition to community engagement is recruiting community champions from the area. This could be anyone interested in being a part of this activity. A good number of our community champions are cancer survivors and women.

4. Garnering philanthropic support

This provides the necessary boost to enhance affordability and accessibility. Bearing in mind that cancer care is expensive and 80% of health care in India continues to be out of pocket, this approach can make a difference.

5. Capacity building

Considering the region's high literacy status, we believed it pragmatic to harness the grassroots-level workers to enhance awareness creation. This led us to prepare training modules for various cadres of the healthcare workforce. The awareness sessions are now spearheaded by trained grassroots-level providers like Accredited Social Health Activists (ASHAs), Anganwadi workers (AWWs), and auxiliary nurse midwives (ANMs). They are supervised by dedicated, trained medical social workers (MSWs). Sessions are also attended by senior community medicine residents so that complex queries could be attended to and myths dispelled. Advanced training sessions in cancer screening and early detection are provided to staff nurses from the government setting to create a larger pool of trained healthcare providers.

6. Creating awareness

Armed with a considerable network of trained individuals, cancer awareness and screening camps are held throughout the year in various parts of the district. Raising awareness is done through a multitude of activities such as street plays, short videos, lectures, games, and quizzes. The community profiling exercises also provide us with the necessary input as to the kind of messages and media that would be received by the people and this aids in customizing the messages accordingly.

SUMMARY

Health promotion strategies aligned with improving the three A's listed next could be a pragmatic model for a diverse country like India with huge disparities:

Factor to be Addressed	**Health Promotion Strategies**		
Awareness	Multiactivity approach	Intersectoral coordination	Customized and targeted approach
Accessibility	Patient advocate	Community participation	Capacity building
Affordability	Philanthropic support	Community participation	Capacity building

REFERENCES

1. Institute for Health Metrics and Evaluation (IHME). *Findings from the Global Burden of Disease Study 2017.* Seattle, WA: IHME, 2018

2. Indian Council of Medical Research (ICMR) (2019). Retrieved from https://www.icmr.nic.in/sites/default/files/ICMR_News_1.pdf

3. Manoharan N, Nair O, Shukla NK, Rath GK. Descriptive epidemiology of female breast cancer in Delhi, India. *Asian Pacific Journal of Cancer Prevention* 2017;18:1015–18. https://doi.org/10.22034/APJCP.2017.18.4.1015

4. Smith RD, Mallath MK. History of the growing burden of cancer in India: From antiquity to the 21st century. *Journal of Global Oncology* 2019;5:1–15. https://doi.org/10.1200/jgo.19.00048

5. Sathwara J, Balasubramaniam G, Bobdey S, Jain A, Saoba S. Sociodemographic factors and late-stage diagnosis of breast cancer in India: A hospital-based study. *Indian Journal of Medical and Paediatric Oncology* 2017;38:277–81. https://doi.org/10.4103/ijmpo.ijmpo_15_16

6. Dwivedi AK, Dwivedi SN, Deo S, Shukla R, Pandey A, Dwivedi DK. An epidemiological study on delay in treatment initiation of cancer patients. *Health* 2012;4:66–79

7. Mallath MK, Taylor DG, Badwe RA, et al. The growing burden of cancer in India: Epidemiology and social context. *Lancet Oncology* 2014;15:e205–e212

8. Nair S, Athreya MR, Kathrikolly T, Kamath A, Vidyasagar MS. Predictors of breast cancer survival in a tertiary care hospital in Coastal Karnataka. *International Journal of Collaborative Research on Internal Medicine & Public Health* 2016;8:45–55

9. Rao RSP, Nair S, Nair NS, Kamath VG. Acceptability and effectiveness of a breast health awareness programme for rural women in India. *Indian Journal of Medical Sciences* 2005;59:398–402. https://doi.org/10.4103/0019-5359.16817

11 Public Health Approaches to Road Traffic Injury Prevention

Geetam Tiwari and Dinesh Mohan

CONTENTS

> A new thinking has evolved about road safety based on accepting that road crashes cannot be avoided (because of human error) and that crashes result from complex combinations of elements that include human behavior, vehicles and infrastructure and need to be addressed by sharing the responsibility for safety between the users and providers of the road transport system.
>
> **World Health Organization, *Preventing Road Traffic Injury: A Public Health Perspective for Europe*, 2004**

ROAD TRAFFIC INJURIES: A PUBLIC HEALTH PROBLEM

Road traffic injuries (RTIs) result from a complex interaction of sociological, psychological, physical, and technological phenomena. Once we accept that traffic injury control is a public health problem, it becomes our ethical responsibility to arrange for the safety of individuals.

The process toward a scientific approach to public health issues is closely related to the historical development of medicine, public health, and epidemiology (Hennekens et al., 1987). The public health approach is a generic analytical framework that has made it possible for different fields of health to respond to a wide range of health problems and diseases, including injuries and violence (Gordon, 1949; Haddon, 1980; Waller, 1989). Disease is the product of the social, economic, and technological environments that people live in. Within this environment, the power to make decisions regarding choices available for one's well-being and the power to influence other people's lives plays an important role in what health benefits are available to society as a whole. This is in line with the World Health Organization's (WHO) definition of health promotion:

> Health promotion enables people to increase control over their health. It covers a wide range of social and environmental interventions that are designed to benefit and protect individual people's health and quality of life by addressing and preventing the root causes of ill health, not just focusing on treatment and cure.*

* https://www.who.int/news-room/q-a-detail/what-is-health-promotion

DOI: 10.1201/b23385-19

The same holds true for traffic injury control and safety promotion. Morbidity and mortality due to traffic injuries have always existed, but their recognition as a public health problem is a phenomenon of the mid-20th century.

When principles of public health are applied to the control of traffic injuries, we can assume the following principles:

- There is no fundamental difference between traffic injuries and the occurrence of any other disease.
- Traffic injury can be defined as a disease that results from an acute exposure of the human body to the transfer of energy from the environment around it.
- "Accidents" and injuries are not "acts of God".
- All injuries cannot be prevented despite our best efforts. This is due to our current knowledge of traffic systems and road users. Therefore, we must be prepared for treating these injuries and their adverse outcomes.

The public health approach to traffic injury prevention involves four interrelated steps:

- The first step is to determine the magnitude, scope, and characteristics of the problem.
- The second step is to identify the factors that increase the risk of disease, injury, or disability, and to determine which factors are potentially modifiable.
- The third step is to assess what measures can be taken to prevent the problem by using the information about causes and risk factors to design, pilot test, and evaluate interventions. This step aims at developing interventions based in large part upon information obtained from the previous steps and testing these or other extant interventions. An important component of the evaluation step is to document the processes that contribute to the success or failure of an intervention in addition to examining the impact of interventions on health outcomes.
- The final step is the implementation of interventions that have been proven or are highly likely to be effective on a broad scale. Another important component is determining the cost-effectiveness of such programs. Balancing the costs of a program against the cases prevented by the intervention can be helpful to policy-makers in determining optimal public health practice. Implementation also implies health communication, and the formation of partnerships and alliances as well as developing methods for community-based programs.

ROAD TRAFFIC INJURY TRENDS: AN INTERNATIONAL COMPARISON

Injuries and deaths due to road traffic crashes have been recognized in the new millennium as a global public health problem by all stakeholders. The WHO released its *World Report on Road Traffic Injury Prevention* in 2004 (Peden et al., 2004). The publication of the report spurred some national and international agencies and civil society groups to give a little more attention to the problem of road safety, and a number of resolutions have been passed by the United Nations General Assembly, World Health Assembly, and the Executive Board of the WHO (WHO, 2004, 2009b, 2011, 2016).

Globally, the number of fatalities per 100,000 persons (mortality rate) ranges from less than 3 to almost 40. The rate is generally less than 9 in high-income countries (HICs) and has a range of 10–40 in low- and middle-income countries (LMICs) with the African region demonstrating the highest average rate of 27 (WHO, 2018). Figure 11.1 shows the trend of death rates due to RTI in nine HICs for 1990–2017. The data show that RTI fatalities per 100,000 persons in all these countries have been declining over this period (Institute for Health Metrics and Evaluation, 2018).

Figure 11.2 shows the Global Burden of Disease 2017 study (Institute for Health Metrics and Evaluation, 2018) estimates for RTI fatality rates for the same period in eight LMICs. These estimates show that death rates are either stable or show some declining trends.

The fatality rates in all these countries are generally greater than 15 per 100,000 persons with South Africa, Malaysia, and Iran having rates as high as 28–30 in 2017. However, the absolute number of fatalities is still increasing in most LMICs because of population increases in these countries. Figure 11.3 shows the total number of RTI fatalities in India from 1970 to 2018. These data indicate that though the total number of fatalities continues to increase in India, the rate per 100,000 persons may not be increasing at the same rate as earlier.

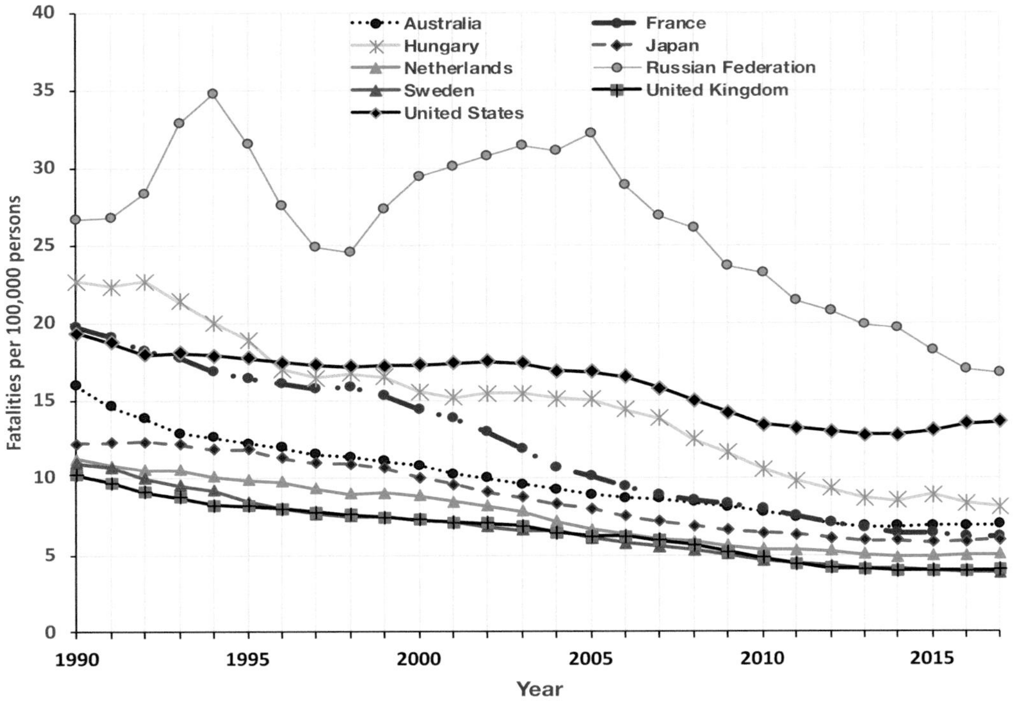

Figure 11.1 Trends in RTI fatality rates in nine high-income countries for 1990–2017. (From Institute for Health Metrics and Evaluation, 2018.)

Road Traffic Injury Patterns in LMICs

With progress made in reducing deaths from communicable diseases, the proportion of deaths from noncommunicable diseases/injuries has increased. It is estimated that, globally, pedestrians and bicyclists comprise 26% of all road traffic deaths and motorized two-wheelers (MTW) comprise 28% (Institute for Health Metrics and Evaluation, 2018).

Traffic crash patterns on LMIC highways are substantially different compared to North America and Western Europe. Pedestrian and motorcyclist involvement in fatal crashes on rural highways is greater than that of other road users. These highway crash patterns are similar to those observed in urban areas. In urban areas, the proportion of people injured "inside the vehicles" is much higher in HICs as compared to LMICs. The number of pedestrians, bicyclists, and MTW users also remains much higher on urban streets in LMICs as compared to HICs.

Road Traffic Injury Data from Asian Countries

Data for the Global Status Reports on Road Safety (GSRRS) 2018 were collected from each participating country, and experts from different sectors within each country completed a self-administered questionnaire with information on key variables. It is widely recognized that fatality statistics suffer from underreporting in many countries and so the WHO team adjusted the fatality figures for a 30-day period for death after the crash. They also used a negative binomial regression model for estimating fatalities for each country by accounting for income, exposure, risk factors, strength of the health system, and other details. Until recently it was not possible to compare RTI trends across countries in Asia, as a majority of them do not use similar definitions and have varied degrees of underreporting. The GSRRS18 has used a scientific approach to estimate the number of RTI fatalities and this makes it possible for us to do some comparisons. In this chapter, we report how the understanding of RTI changes if we analyze the GSRRS18 estimates and compare them with self-reported statistics from different countries.

A summary of the data reported for 27 Asian countries is given in Table 11.1. These data show that 11 countries (41%) were not able to supply complete data on the proportion of different types of road users killed in crashes.

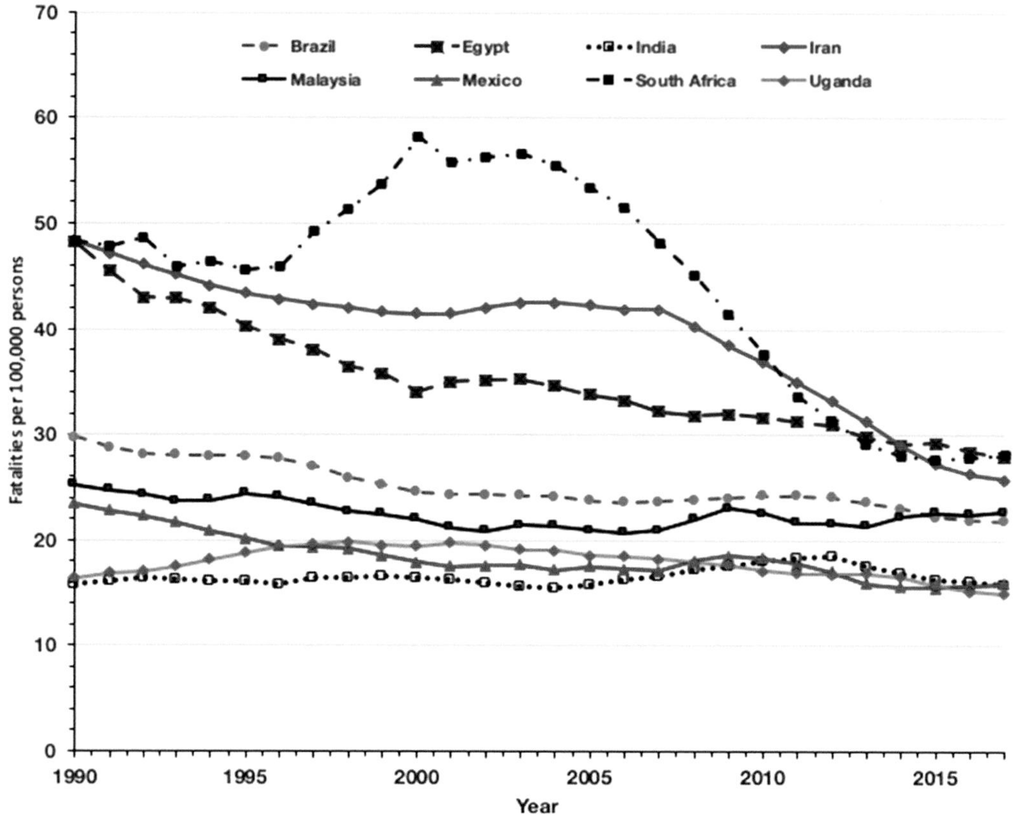

Figure 11.2 Trends in RTI fatality rates in eight low- and middle-income countries for 1990–2017. (From Institute for Health Metrics and Evaluation, 2018.)

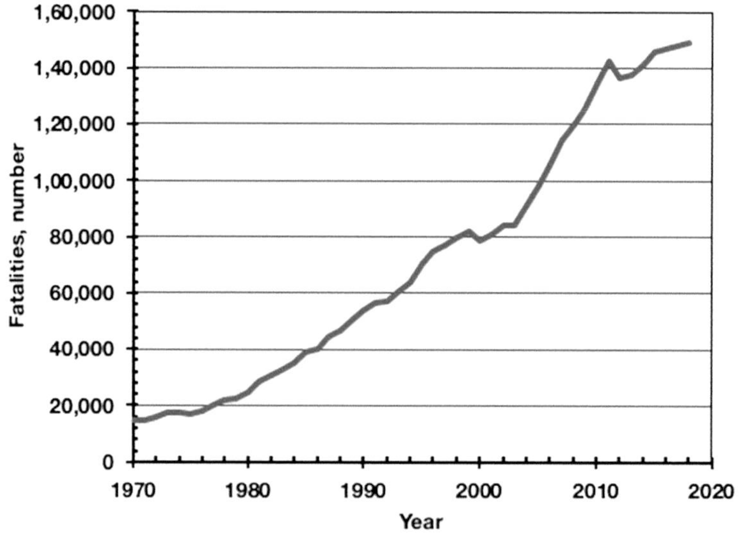

Figure 11.3 Number of people killed in road traffic crashes in India from 1970 to 2018. (From Ministry of Road Transport and Highways, Government of India.)

Table 11.1: Road Traffic Injury Statistics for Selected Asian Countries

Country	Population 2016	GNI per capita USS 2016	Deaths per 100,000 persons		Reported rate/ WHO rate	Occupant deaths percent				
			Country reported data	WHO estimate		Drivers/ Passengers 4 wheeled vehicles	Drivers / Passengers 2- or 3- wheelers	Cyclists	Pedestrians	Other/ unspecified
Afghanistan	34,656,032	580	4.5	15.1	0.30	—	—	—	—	—
Bangladesh	162,951,552	1,330	1.5	15.3	0.10	—	—	—	—	—
Bhutan	797,765	2,510	15.7	17.4	0.90	—	—	—	—	—
Cambodia	15,762,370	1,140	1 1.7	17.8	0.66	6.2	73.5	2.3	9.6	8.4
China	1,411,415,375	8,260	4.1	18.2	0.23	—	—	—	—	—
India	1,324,171,392	1,680	1 1.4	22.6	0.50	17.9	39.6	1.7	10.4	30.4
Indonesia	261,1 15,456	3,400	12.0	12.2	0.99	4.9	73.6	3.2	15.5	2.7
Iran	80,277,424	6,530	19.8	20.5	0.97	48.7	24.1	0.6	21.6	5
Japan	127,748,512	38,000	3.7	4.1	0.90	32.4	17.2	15.1	35	1
Jordan	9,455,802	3,920	7.9	24.4	0.33	71.3	0	0	28.7	0
Kuwait	4,052,584	4 1,680	10.5	17.6	0.59	—	—	—	—	—
Lao PDR	6,758,353	2,150	16.1	16.6	0.97	—	—	—	—	—
Malaysia	31,187,264	9,850	22.9	23.6	0.97	—	—	—	—	—
Maldives	427,756	7,430	0.9	0.9	1.00	0	75	0	25	0
Myanmar	52,885,224	1,190	9.2	19.9	0.46	10.8	64.8	3.1	14.2	7.1
Nepal	28,982,772	730	6.9	15.9	0.43	—	—	—	—	—
Oman	4,424,762	18,080	15.6	16.1	0.97	64.7	3.9	0.7	22.5	8.1
Pakistan	193,203,472	1,510	2.3	14.3	0.16	—	—	—	—	—
Philippines	103,320,224	3,580	9.7	12.3	0.79	0.3	4.7	0.1	1	93.9
Qatar	2,569,804	75,660	6.9	9.3	0.74	48.3	2.2	2.8	32	14.6
R. of Korea	50,791,920	27,600	8.5	9.8	0.86	—	20.5	5.9	39.9	33.7
Saudi Arabia	32,275,688	21,750	28.0	28.8	0.97	—	—	—	—	—
Singapore	5,622,455	51,880	2.5	2.8	0.91	7.8	44	14.2	33.3	0.7
Sri Lanka	20,798,492	3,780	14.4	14.9	0.97	6.2	50.8	8.1	29.2	5.7
Thailand	68,863,512	5,640	31.6	32.7	0.97	12.3	74.4	3.5	7.6	2.3
UAE	9,269,612	40,480	7.8	18.1	0.43	54.5	5.5	1.5	24.3	14.2
Viet Nam	94,569,072	2,050	8.9	26.4	0.34	—	—	—	—	—

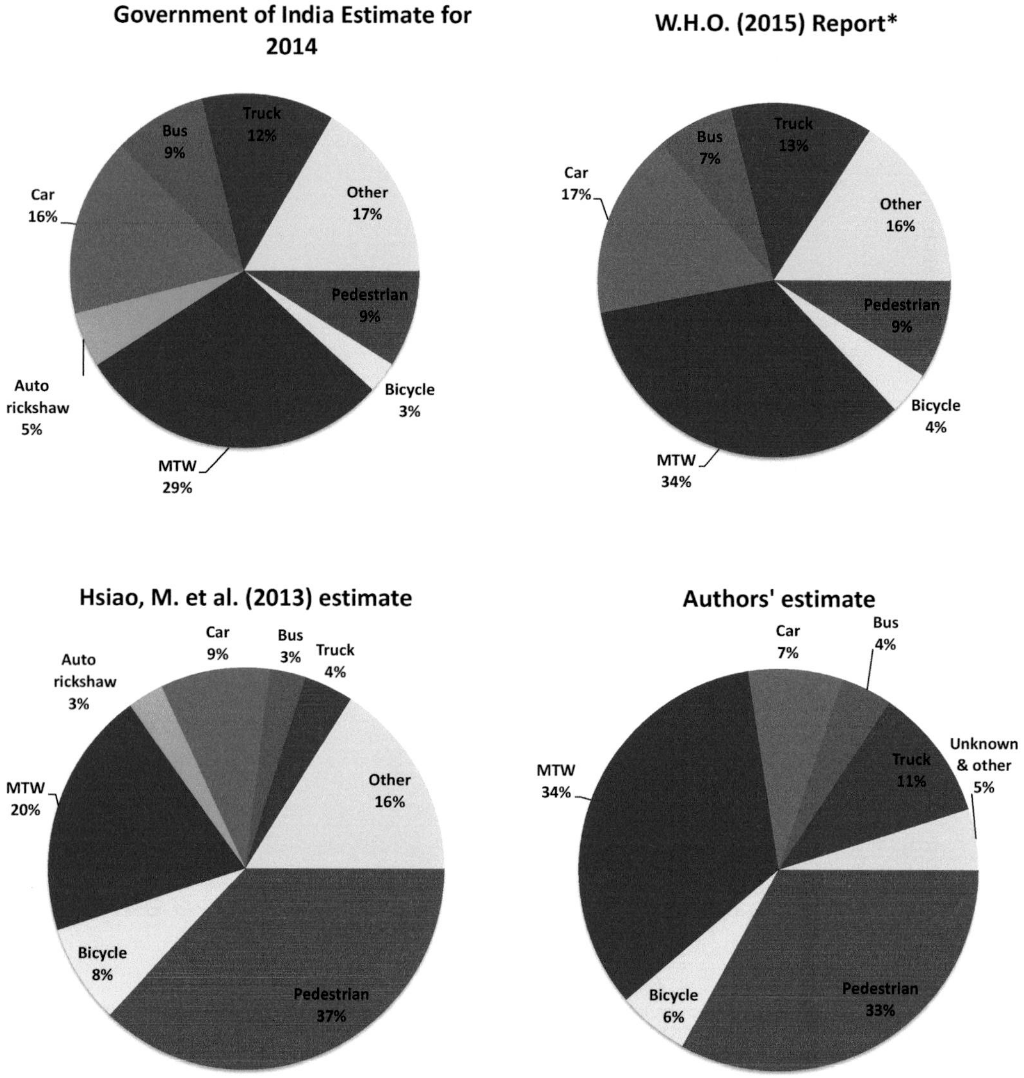

Figure 11.4 Estimates of the share of different road user fatalities in India. (From Transport Research Wing, 2017; Hsiao et al., 2013; Institute for Health Metrics and Evaluation, 2018; Mohan et al., 2017.)

Data from different studies for fatalities by different road-user types in India are given in Figure 11.4. The data included in the WHO report indicate that the proportion of four-wheeler occupants killed in India is greater than that of pedestrians or bicyclists, and the other/unspecified proportion is 30%. The in-depth studies conducted in India show a much higher proportion of vulnerable road users killed in cities and highways (Hsiao et al., 2013; Mohan et al., 2017; Transport Research Wing, 2017). This difference is explained by the fact that the data submitted for India is partly based on official national statistics reported for fatalities by vehicle type (NCRB, 2015). In the Government of India's reports, the vehicle type is probably recorded as the one that was thought to be at fault and not the one in which the victim was traveling. This is the reason that bicyclists and pedestrians have low proportions in the Indian government and WHO reports. This analysis for India illustrates the problems faced in collecting reliable traffic injury data from around the world.

Figure 11.5 shows the country-reported data and WHO estimates for RTI fatality rates per 100,000 persons plotted against national per-capita income (WHO, 2015). Only 10 (37%) of the countries reported fatality rates close to the WHO estimates. The WHO estimates for fatalities in India

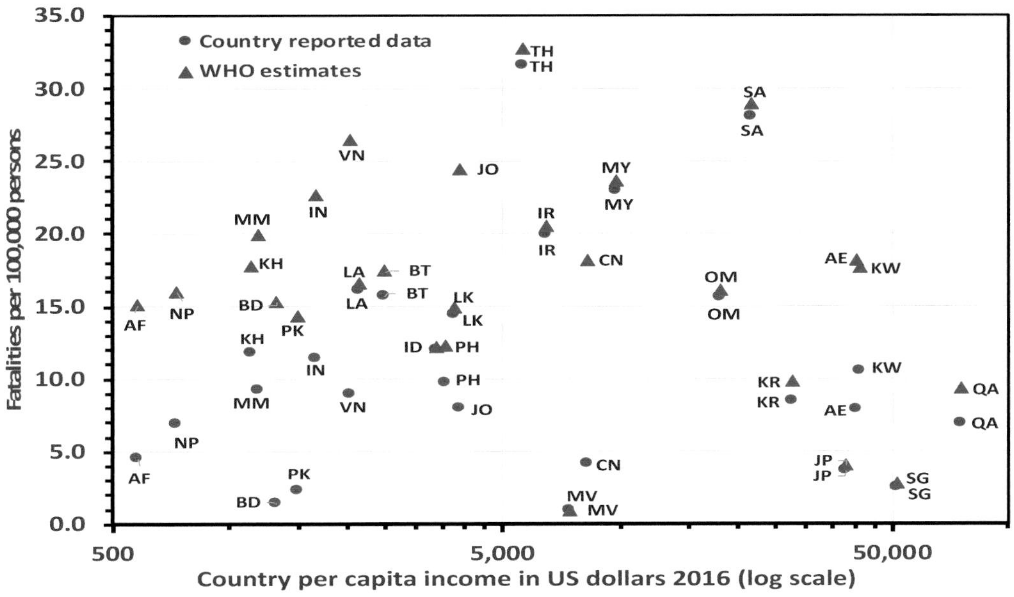

Figure 11.5 Road traffic fatality rates for Asian countries versus national per capita income. (From WHO, 2018.) Two letter codes in the chart denote countries listed in the chapter Appendix.

is 50% greater than the reported fatality rate. It is widely recognized that the official estimates for road traffic fatalities can be underestimates (Jacobs et al., 2000). While more high-income countries seem to have reported rates closer to WHO estimates than low-income countries, it is interesting that both low-income and high-income countries can have underreporting and realistic reporting. Even if the estimates do not reflect the reality accurately, they do reflect the extent of underreporting. However, it appears that is not necessary to have high-income levels to develop reliable RTI reporting systems as commonly assumed.

Figure 11.5 also shows that national RTI fatality rates per 100,000 persons as reported by countries nor WHO estimates have a high correlation with national per capita income in Asia. The WHO estimates seem to have a lower correlation with income than the rates reported by individual countries. Some HICs such as the United Arab Emirates (AE), Kuwait (KW), and Saudi Arabia (SA) have higher rates than LMICs like Indonesia (ID) and the Philippines (PH). This suggests that higher national incomes do not necessarily produce better road safety policies. This is contrary to the widely held belief that RTI rates are highly dependent on per-capita incomes (Kopits & Cropper, 2005). Figure 11.6 shows that, in general, countries that have a higher proportion of two- or three-wheel vehicles in their fleet have a higher proportion of two- or three-wheeler occupant fatalities (WHO, 2009a). However, there is a reasonable spread of fatality proportions for each vehicle proportion. Japan (JP) and Singapore (SG) are HICs that have similar two- or three-wheeler fleet ratios (reporting is likely to be reliable; country and WHO fatality estimates are similar) but Singapore's fatality ratio is 2.7 times greater than that of Japan though its overall fatality rates are similar. This indicates that even countries that have similar incomes, vehicle fleet ratios, motor vehicle standards, and traffic regulations can have different fatality patterns. This is probably due to other factors influencing fatality rates, such as urban living patterns, and street and highway infrastructure (Mohan et al., 2017).

Figure 11.6 shows that this is only roughly true and generally car proportions increase and two- or three-wheeler proportions decrease with increases in per-capita incomes. (The numbers do not add up to 100 for each country, as other vehicles are not included.) However, there are large variations at similar levels of income. The correlation by income is weak for country incomes less than $10,000 per capita. Since most Asian countries are below US$10,000 income levels at present, it is unlikely that many countries' annual per-capita incomes will exceed US$10,000 in the next two decades. At present, Japan is the only HIC in Asia with a large population. Therefore, we are likely to see continuing high use of MTWs in most Asian countries.

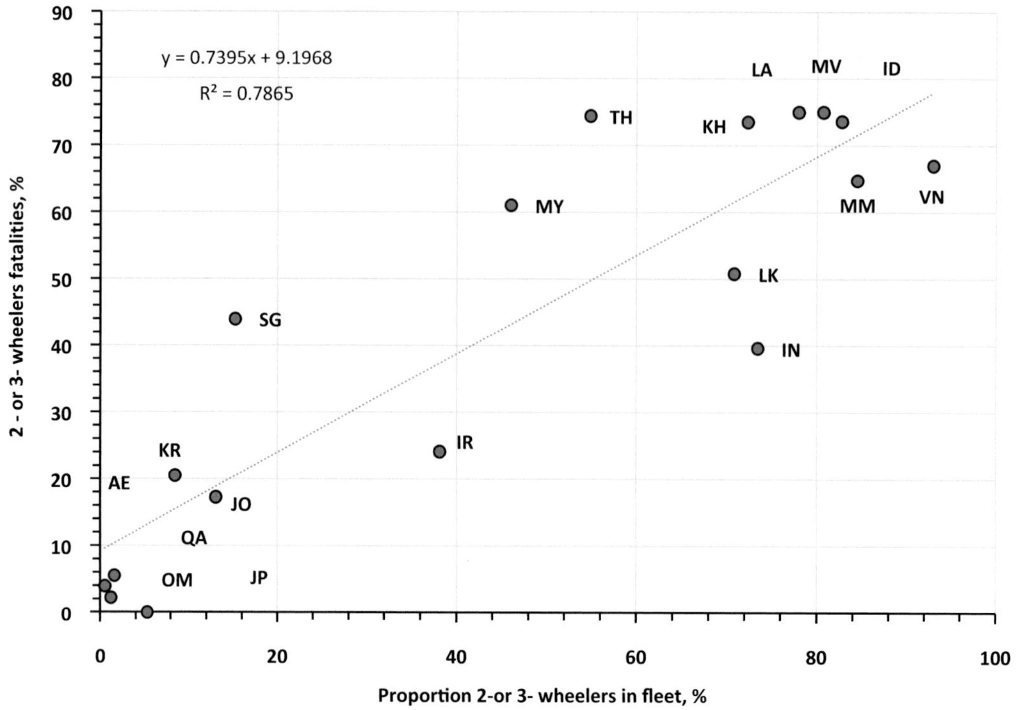

Figure 11.6 Proportion of two- or three-wheeler occupant fatalities versus the proportion of two- or three-wheeled vehicles in the country fleet. (From Olson et al., 2016; WHO, 2018.) The two-letter codes in the chart denote countries listed in the chapter Appendix.

OUR UNDERSTANDING OF THE SCIENCE OF TRAFFIC INJURIES

Safety science has influenced traffic safety interventions in HICs. Starting with the recognition of injury as a disease in the mid-20th century, many researchers adopted the public health approach to suggest road safety interventions. This led to the emergence of the safe systems approach in the Netherlands and Vision Zero in Sweden.

Research has established that the principal cause of why people die and are seriously injured is that the energy to which people are exposed in a traffic accident is excessive in relation to the energy that the human frame can withstand. Knowledge of energy and tolerance has to a great extent served as a basis for the development we have seen of the passive safety characteristics of vehicles and for the development of different protection systems such as child safety seats, helmets, and seat belts. Speed is an important factor affecting road accidents both in terms of accident occurrence and severity. It seems reasonably safe to assume that increased speed would mean that the accidents that have occurred would be more severe if other factors (e.g., environment and vehicle design) remain the same. A large number of studies have shown this by both Newtonian physics and empirical data.

Learnings from Scientific Research

International road safety research has involved a large number of very well-trained professionals from a variety of disciplines over the past four decades. Some very innovative work has resulted in a theoretical understanding of road traffic crashes as a part of a complex interaction of sociological, psychological, physical, and technological phenomena. This understanding of injuries and crashes has helped high-income countries design safer vehicles, roads, and traffic management systems. A similar effort for research, development, and innovation is needed in India and similar countries. A much larger group of committed professionals and multidisciplinary stakeholders needs to be involved in this work for new ideas to emerge.

RESULTS OF SYSTEMATIC REVIEWS

Legislation and Enforcement

Legislation can be a very strong policy instrument to promote traffic safety. There are many examples of major changes in road-user behavior and accidents associated with the introduction of new legislation. Laws do not enforce themselves. Laws are to be enforced to encourage safe behavior from road users. Enforcement is therefore very important for maintaining the effects of laws.

Increased normal, stationary speed enforcement is in most cases cost-effective. Automatic speed enforcement seems to be even more efficient. However, there is no evidence to prove that mobile traffic enforcement for speed control with patrol cars is cost-effective (Carlsson, 1997).

The only effective way to get most motorists to use safety belts is with laws requiring their use and sustained enforcement. When laws are in place, education and/or advertising can be used to inform the public about the laws and their enforcement (O'Neill, 2001).

In general, the deterrent effect of a law is determined in part by the swiftness and visibility of the penalty for disobeying the law, but a key factor is the perceived likelihood of being detected and sanctioned. Laws against drinking and driving are effective when combined with active enforcement and the support of the community (Elder et al., 2004; Koornstra, 2007; Sweedler et al., 2004).

Education Campaigns and Driver Education

Road safety campaigns often aim to improve road-user behavior by increasing knowledge and by changing attitudes. There is no clearly proven relationship between knowledge and attitudes on the one hand and behavior on the other (O'Neill, 2001; OECD, 1986). Most highway safety educational programs do not work. They do not reduce motor vehicle crash deaths and injuries (Robertson, 1980, 1983; Robertson et al., 1974). Only a few programs have ever been shown to work, and contrary to the view that education cannot do any harm, some programs have been shown to make matters worse (Robertson, 1980; Sandels, 1975).

Driver or pedestrian education programs by themselves usually are insufficient to reduce crash rates (Elvik & Vaa, 2004). They may increase knowledge and even induce some behavior change, but this does not seem to result in a reduction in crash rates (Duperrex, Roberts, & Bunn, 2003; Roberts et al., 2003). There is, however, no reason to waste money on general campaigns. Campaigns should be used to put important questions on the agenda, and campaigns aimed at changing road-user behavior should be focused on clearly defined behaviors and should by preference fortify other measures such as new legislation and/or police enforcement.

The effects of campaigns using tangible incentives (rewards) to promote safety-belt usage have been evaluated using a meta-analytical approach. The results (weighted mean effect) show a mean short-term increase in use rates of 12.0 percentage points; the mean long-term effect was 9.6 percentage points (Hagenzieker et al., 1997).

Studies show that driver education may be necessary for beginners to learn the elementary skills for obtaining a license, but compulsory training in schools leads to early licensing. There is no evidence that driver education in schools results in a reduction in road crash rates. On the other hand, they may lead to increased road crash rates (Mayhew et al., 1998; Vernick et al., 1999; Williams & O'Neill, 1974). While there may be a need to train professional drivers in the use of heavy vehicles, there is no evidence that formal driver education should be compulsory in schools and colleges.

Compulsory helmet use reduces bicycle-related head and facial injuries for bicyclists of all ages involved in all types of crashes, including those involving motor vehicles (Thompson et al., 1999). Similar results have been confirmed for motorcyclists (American College of Surgeons, 2001; Bledsoe et al., 2002; Brandt et al., 2002; Liu et al., 2003; McKnight & McKnight, 1995; Mohan et al., 1984; National Highway Traffic Safety, 1996).

Vehicle Factors

Vehicles conforming to European Union or US crashworthiness standards provide significant safety benefits to occupants and the effectiveness of the following measures have been evaluated.

The use of seat belts and airbag-equipped cars can reduce car-occupant fatalities by over 30%. It is estimated that airbag deployment reduced mortality by 63%, while lap–shoulder belt use reduced mortality by 72%, and combined airbag and seat belt use reduced mortality by more than 80% (Crinion et al., 1975; Kent et al., 2005; Parkin et al., 1993). High-mounted rear brake lights reduce the incidence of rear-end crashes (ETSC, 1993) (Figure 11.7).

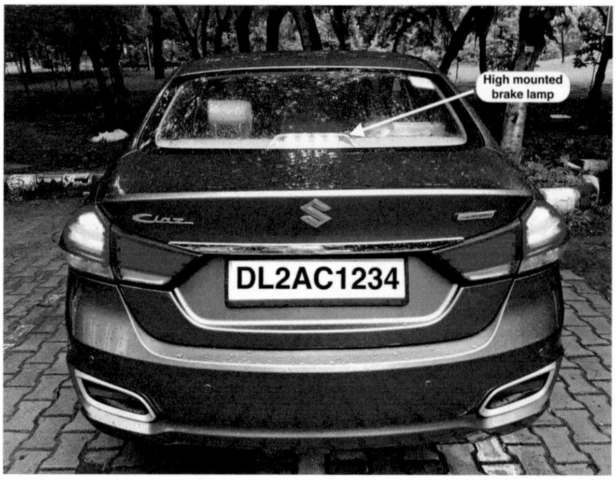

Figure 11.7 High-mounted brake lamps in cars.

Improvements in vehicle crashworthiness and restraint use have contributed to a major reduction in occupant fatality rates and are estimated to be more than 40% in most reviews (Elvik & Vaa, 2004; Koornstra, 2007; Noland, 2003).

Alcohol locks are technologies that could prevent a vehicle from being driven when the device registers that the driver's blood alcohol concentration (BAC) exceeds the legal limit prevalent in the country. These technologies range from relatively simple ones where the driver is required to blow into an alcohol testing unit before starting the car to more sophisticated ones that sense the presence of alcohol in the air and in the bloodstream of the driver (Zaouk et al., 2015).

Environmental and Infrastructure Factors

The environment and geometric features of the road (horizontal and vertical curves, median design, shoulder width, etc.) directly affect road-user behavior. Straight wide lanes encourage high-speed driving and drivers are likely to exceed speed limits. On the other hand, narrow lanes discourage high-speed driving. A lack of service roads often results in slow-moving nonmotorized traffic occupying the left lane next to high-speed traffic. Also, raised medians result in overturned-vehicle crashes. Therefore, the road environment and infrastructure must be adapted to the limitations of the road users (Van Vliet & Schermers, 2000). In case the driver makes a mistake and hits the median or goes off the main carriageway, the median design should be able to contain the vehicle without causing harm to the vehicle occupant.

Traffic-calming techniques, use of roundabouts, and provision of bicycle facilities in urban areas provide significant safety benefits, and limited-access highways with appropriate shoulder and median designs provide significant safety benefits on long-distance roads (Elvik, 1995, 2001; Hyden & Varhelyi, 2000). Though improvements in road design seem to have some beneficial effects on crash rates, increases in speed and exposure can offset some of these benefits (Noland, 2003; O'Neill & Kyrychenko, 2006). Therefore, additional measures may be required to manage safe speeds.

Road designs that control speed seem to be the most effective crash control measures (Aarts & Van Schagen, 2006). A great deal of additional work needs to be done on rural and urban roads and infrastructure design suitable for mixed traffic to make the environment safer for vulnerable road users. This would require special guidelines and standards for the design of (a) roundabouts, (b) service lanes along all intercity highways, and (c) traffic calming on urban roads and highways passing through settlements.

POLICY FRAMEWORK AND RECOMMENDED STRATEGIES

A study of the international literature on how countries have improved their safety performance over the years shows a multitude of potential explanations. In the last few decades, traffic safety measures have been focused on (1) improving human behavior (speed, alcohol, seat belts, and helmets) through legislation, enforcement, and campaigns; (2) safer infrastructure through planning and design; and (3) safer vehicles through better crashworthiness and active vehicle safety.

Internationally, three important principles have been accepted for promoting road safety strategies: (1) a road environment with an infrastructure adapted to the limitations of the road user; (2) vehicles equipped with technology to simplify the driving task and with features that protect vulnerable and other road users; and (3) road users that are well informed and adequately educated. The basic premise behind these principles is the acceptance of the limitations of road users, such as impatient pedestrians, a risk-taking attitude among young drivers, and bicyclists and pedestrians always looking for paths that are short and require little effort. The road environment must be designed in such a way that despite these limitations, the probability of injury and severity of injury can be reduced.

Pedestrian and Bicyclist Safety

1. Reserving adequate space for nonmotorized modes on all urban roads and highways near urban areas (Figure 11.8).
2. Appropriate design of roundabouts along with raised pedestrian crossings in urban areas.
3. Free left turns must be banned at all signalized intersections. This will give a safe time for pedestrians and bicyclists to cross the road.
4. Maximum speed limits of 40–50 km/h on arterial roads need to be enforced by road design and police monitoring in urban areas. Maximum speeds of 30 km/h in residential areas need to be enforced by judicious use of speed bumps and mini roundabouts.
5. Increasing the conspicuousness of bicycles by fixing reflectors on all sides and wheels, and painting them yellow, white, or orange (Figure 11.9).

Motorcyclist and Motor Vehicle Safety

1. Notification of mandatory use of helmet and daytime headlights by two-wheeler riders.
2. All cars should conform to the latest international crashworthiness regulations.
3. Pedestrian safety regulations for car drivers to be notified.
4. Enforce seatbelt-use laws countrywide.
5. Restricting front-seat travel in cars by children and the use of child seats has the potential for reducing injuries to child occupants.
6. Introduction of active safety technologies like automatic braking, pedestrian detection, electronic stability control, and alcohol locks.

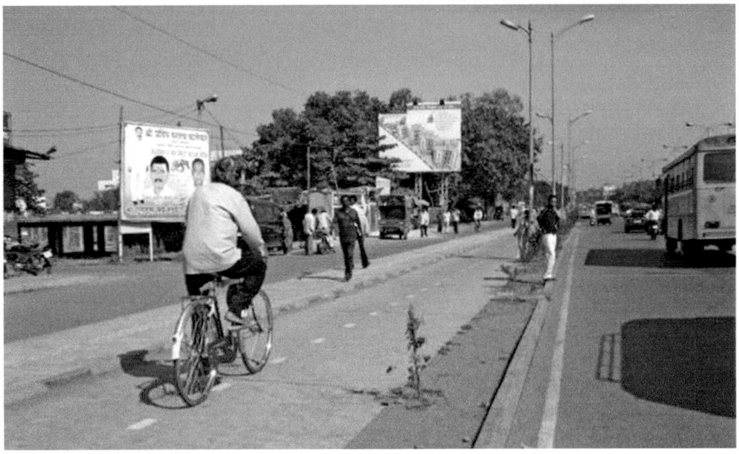

Figure 11.8 Segregated cycle track on Solapur Road, Pune.

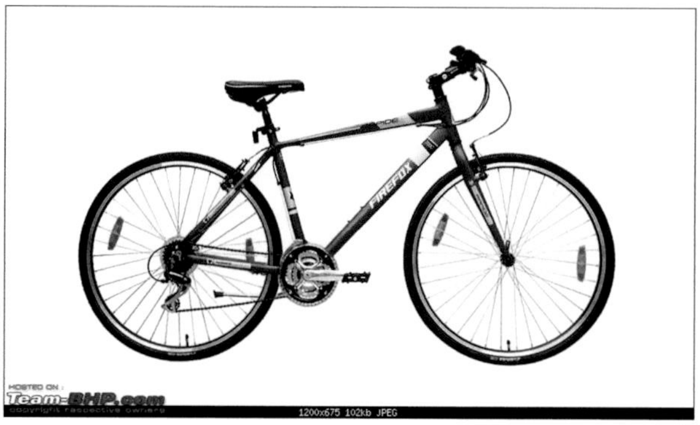

Figure 11.9 Bicycle with reflectors.

Road Measures

1. Support traffic calming in urban areas and on rural highways passing through towns and villages.
2. Improve existing traffic circles by bringing them in accordance with modern roundabout practices and substituting existing signalized intersections with roundabouts.
3. Provide provision of segregated bicycle lanes and disability-friendly pedestrian paths.
4. Require mandatory road safety audits for all road building and improvement projects.
5. Construct service lanes along all four-lane highways and expressways for use by low-speed and nonmotorized traffic.
6. Remove raised medians (center medians) on intercity highways and replace them with steel guard rails or wire rope barriers.
7. Install appropriate crash barriers on all high-speed roads on the edge of the shoulder.

Enforcement

1. The most important enforcement issue in India is speed control. Without this, it will be difficult to lower crash rates, as a majority of the victims are vulnerable road users.
2. The second most important measure to be taken seriously is driving under the influence of alcohol. About 30%–40% of fatal crashes in India may have alcohol involvement.
3. Enforce seat belt and helmet use.

Prehospital Care, Treatment, and Rehabilitation

1. Modern knowledge regarding prehospital care should be made widely available with the training of specialists in trauma care in the hospital setting.
2. Prehospital care programs should be rationalized on evidence-based policies so that scarce resources are not wasted.

Research Agenda

1. Develop street designs and traffic-calming measures that suit mixed traffic with a high proportion of motorcycles and nonmotorized modes.
2. Design highways with adequate and safe facilities for slow traffic.
3. Design lighter helmets with ventilation.
4. Review pedestrian impact standards for small cars, buses, and trucks.
5. Evaluate policing techniques to minimize cost and maximize effectiveness.

6. Investigate the effectiveness of prehospital care measures.
7. Study traffic-calming measures for mixed traffic streams, including the high proportion of motorized two-wheelers.

Institutional Arrangements

International experience suggests that unless a country establishes an independent national road traffic safety agency it is almost impossible to promote safety in a comprehensive and scientific manner. This was stated powerfully in the report *Reducing Traffic Injury: A Global Challenge* almost 22 years ago (Trinca et al., 1988):

> Each country should create (where one does not exist) a separate traffic safety agency with sufficient executive power and funding to enable meaningful choices between strategy and program options. Such an agency would ideally report directly to the main legislative/political forum or the head of government.

The World Health Organization, in its *World Report on Road Traffic Injury Prevention* (Peden et al., 2004), recommends the following:

1. Make road safety a political priority.
2. Appoint a lead agency for road safety, give it adequate resources, and make it publicly accountable.
3. Develop a multidisciplinary approach to road safety.
4. Set appropriate road safety targets and establish national road safety plans to achieve them.
5. Create budgets for road safety and increase investment in demonstrably effective road safety activities.

In India, the Ministry of Roads and Highways is responsible for monitoring road safety. After a decade-long discussion for establishing a road safety agency in India, the Motor Vehicle Act was amended in 2019, which suggested:

> (1) The Central Government shall, by notification in the Official Gazette, constitute a National Road Safety Board consisting of a Chairman, such number of representatives from the State Governments, and such other members as it may consider necessary and on such terms and conditions as may be prescribed by the Central Government. (2) The National Board shall render advice to the Central Government or State Government, as the case may be, on all aspects pertaining to road safety and traffic management.

A National Road Safety Board has not been established so far. The Supreme Court, via an order dated 22 April 2014 in Writ Petition (C) No 295 of 2012, constituted a committee under the chairmanship of Justice KS Radhakrishnan, to measure and monitor on behalf of the court the implementation of various laws relating to road, vehicles, and trauma care. The committee is pursuing with the states to ensure that they regularly hold meetings of the district road safety committee (DRSC) and also monitor their performance in order to reduce road accidents and fatalities.

REFERENCES

Aarts, L., & Van Schagen, I. (2006). Driving speed and the risk of road crashes: A review. *Accident Analysis & Prevention, 38*(2), 215–224.

American College of Surgeons. (2001). Statement in support of motorcycle helmet laws [ST-35]. *Bulletin of the American College of Surgeons, 86*(2).

Bledsoe, G. H., Schexnayder, S. M., Carey, M. J., Dobbins, W. N., Gibson, W. D., Hindman, J. W., … & Ferrer, T. J. (2002). The negative impact of the repeal of the Arkansas motorcycle helmet law. *Journal of Trauma, 53*(6), 1078–1086.

Brandt, M. M., Ahrns, K. S., Corpron, C. A., Franklin, G. A., & Wahl, W. L. (2002). Hospital cost is reduced by motorcycle helmet use. *Journal of Trauma, 53*(3), 469–471.

Carlsson, G. (1997). Cost-effectiveness of information, campaigns and enforcement and the costs and benefits of speed changes. European Seminar on Cost-Effectiveness of Road Safety Work and Measures, Luxembourg.

Crinion, J. D., Foldvary, L. A., & Lane, J. C. (1975). The effect on casualties of a compulsory seat belt wearing law in South Australia. *Accident Analysis & Prevention, 7*(2), 81–89.

Elder, R. W., Shults, R. A., Sleet, D. A., Nichols, J. L., Thompson, R. S., & Rajab, W. (2004). Effectiveness of mass media campaigns for reducing drinking and driving and alcohol-involved crashes: A systematic review. *American Journal of Preventive Medicine, 27*(1), 57–65.

Elvik, R. (1995). The safety value of guardrails and crash cushions: A meta-analysis of evidence from evaluation studies. *Accident Analysis & Prevention, 27*(4), 523–549.

Elvik, R. (2001). Area-wide urban traffic calming schemes: A meta-analysis of safety effects. *Accident Analysis & Prevention, 33*(3), 327–336.

Elvik, R., & Vaa, T. (2004). *The Handbook of Road Safety Measures.* Amsterdam: Elsevier.

ETSC. (1993). *Reducing Traffic Injuries Through Vehicle Safety Improvements.* Brussels: ETSC.

Gordon, J. E. (1949). The epidemiology of accidents. *American Journal of Public Health and the Nation's Health, 39*(4), 504–515. doi:10.2105/AJPH.39.4.504

Haddon, W., Jr. (1980). Advances in the epidemiology of injuries as a basis for public policy. *Public Health Reports, 95*(5), 411–421.

Hagenzieker, M. P., Bijleveld, F. D., & Davidse, R. J. (1997). Effects of incentive programs to stimulate safety belt use: A meta-analysis. *Accident Analysis and Prevention, 29*(6), 759–777.

Hennekens, C. H., Buring, J. E., Mayrent, S. L., & Doll, R. (1987). *Epidemiology in Medicine.* Boston, MA: Little, Brown.

Hsiao, M., Malhotra, A., Thakur, J., Sheth, J. K., Nathens, A. B., Dhingra, N., … & Collaborators, M. D. S. (2013). Road traffic injury mortality and its mechanisms in India: Nationally representative mortality survey of 1.1 million homes. *BMJ Open, 3*(8), e002621.

Hyden, C., & Varhelyi, A. (2000). The effects on safety, time consumption and environment of large scale use of roundabouts in an urban area: A case study. *Accident Analysis & Prevention, 32*(1), 11–23.

Institute for Health Metrics and Evaluation. (2018). *Global Burden of Disease Study 2017 (GBD 2017) Results.* Seattle, WA: IMHE. Retrieved from https://http://vizhub.healthdata.org/gbd-compare/

Jacobs, G., Aeron-Thomas, A., & Astrop, A. (2000). *Estimating Global Road Fatalities.* Crowthorne: TRL.

Kent, R., Viano, D. C., & Crandall, J. (2005). The field performance of frontal air bags: A review of the literature. *Traffic Injury Prevention, 6*(1), 1–23.

Koornstra, M. (2007). Prediction of traffic fatalities and prospects for mobility becoming sustainable-safe. *Sadhna: Academy Proceedings in Engineering Sciences, 32*(4), 365–396.

Kopits, E., & Cropper, M. (2005). Traffic fatalities and economic growth. *Accident Analysis & Prevention, 37*(1), 169–178.

Liu, B., Ivers, R., Norton, R., Blows, S., & Lo, S. K. (2003). Helmets for preventing injury in motorcycle riders (Publication no. 10.1002/14651858.CD004333.pub2). From *Cochrane Database of Systematic Reviews, 2003*. https://doi.org/10.1002/14651858.CD004333.pub2

Mayhew DR, Simpson HM, Williams AF, Ferguson SA. Effectiveness and role of driver education and training in a graduated licensing system. *Journal of Public Health Policy*, 1998;*19*(1):51–67.

McKnight, A. J., & McKnight, A. S. (1995). The effects of motorcycle helmets upon seeing and hearing. *Accident Analysis & Prevention*, *27*(4), 493–501.

Mohan, D., Bangdiwala, S. I., & Villaveces, A. (2017). Urban street structure and traffic safety. *Journal of Safety Research*, *62*, 63–71. https://doi.org/10.1016/j.jsr.2017.06.003

Mohan, D., Kothiyal, K. P., Misra, B. K., & Banerji, A. K. (1984). Helmet and head injury study of crash involved motorcyclists in Delhi. Proceedings 1984 International Conference on the Biomechanics of Impacts (pp. 65–77). Bron, France: IRCOBI.

Mohan, D., Tiwari, G., & Bhalla, K. (2017). *Road Safety in India: Status Report 2016*. New Delhi: TRIPP, IIT Delhi.

National Highway Traffic Safety Administration (1996). *Do Motorcycle Helmets Interfere With the Vision and Hearing of Riders?* Washington, DC: NHTSA.

NCRB (2015). *Accidental Deaths and Suicides in India 2014*. New Delhi: NCRB.

Noland, R. B. (2003). Traffic fatalities and injuries: The effect of changes in infrastructure and other trends. *Accident Analysis & Prevention*, *35*(4), 599–612.

O'Neill, B. (2001). Role of advocacy, education, and training in reducing motor vehicle crash losses. Proceedings from WHO Meeting to Develop a 5-Year Strategy on Road Traffic Injury Prevention. Geneva: WHO.

O'Neill, B., & Kyrychenko, S. (2006). *Use and Misuse of Motor Vehicle Crash Death Rates in Assessing Highway Safety Performance*. Arlington, VA: IIHS.

OECD. (1986). *OECD Road Safety Research: A Synthesis*. Paris: OECD.

Parkin, S., MacKay, G. M., & Framton, R. I. (1993). Effectiveness and limitations of current seat belts in Europe. *Chronic Diseases in Canada*, *14*(4 Supplement), S53–S59.

Peden, M., Scurfield, R., Sleet, D., Mohan, D., Hyder, A. A., Jarawan, E., & Mathers, C. (2004). *World Report on Road Traffic Injury Prevention*. Geneva: WHO.

Roberts, I. G., & Kwan, I. (2001). School-based driver education for the prevention of traffic crashes. *Cochrane Database of Systematic Reviews, 3*. https://doi.org/10.1002/14651858.CD003201

Robertson, L. S. (1980). Crash involvement of teenaged drivers when driver education is eliminated from high school. *American Journal of Public Health*, *70*(6), 599–603.

Robertson, L. S. (1983). *Injuries: Causes, Control Strategies and Public Policy*. Lexington, MA: Lexington Books.

Robertson, L. S., Kelley, A. B., O'Neill, B., Wixom, C. W., Eiswirth, R. S., & Haddon, W., Jr. (1974). A controlled study of the effect of television messages on safety belt use. *American Journal of Public Health*, *64*(11), 1071–1080.

Sandels, S. (1975). *Children in Traffic*. Surrey: Elek Books Ltd.

Sweedler, B., Biecheler, M., Laurell, H., Kroj, G., Lerner, M., Mathijssen, M., … & Tunbridge, R. (2004). Worldwide trends in alcohol and drug impaired driving. *Traffic Injury Prevention, 5*(3), 175–184.

Roberts, I. G., & Kwan, I. (2001). School-based driver education for the prevention of traffic crashes. *Cochrane Database of Systematic Reviews, 3*. https://doi.org/10.1002/14651858.CD003201

Thompson, D. C., Rivara, F., & Thompson, R. (1999). Helmets for preventing head and facial injuries in bicyclists. *Cochrane Database of Systematic Reviews*, 4. doi:10.1002/14651858.CD001855

Transport Research Wing. (2017). *Road Accidents in India: 2016*. New Delhi: Jam Nagar House.

Trinca, G. W., Johnston, I. R., Campbell, B. J., Haight, F. A., Knight, P. R., MacKay, G. M., … & Petrucelli, E. (1988). *Reducing Traffic Injury: A Global Challenge*. Melbourne: Royal Australasian College of Surgeons.

Van Vliet, P., & Schermers, G. (2000). *Sustainable Safety: A New Approach for Road Safety in the Netherlands*. Rotterdam: Traffic Research Centre, Ministry of Transport.

Vernick, J. S., Guohua, L., Ogaitis, S., MacKenzie, E. J., Baker, S. P., & Gielen, A. C. (1999). Effects of high school driver education on motor vehicle crashes, violations, and licensure. *American Journal of Preventive Medicine, 16*(Supplement), 40–46.

Waller, J. A. (1989). Injury control in perspective. *American Journal of Public Health, 79*(3), 272–273.

WHO. (2004). *Road Safety and Health: Resolution WHA57.10*. Retrieved from Geneva: http://www.who.int/roadsafety/about/resolutions/download/en/

WHO. (2009a). *Global Status Report on Road Safety: Time for Action*. Geneva: World Health Organization.

WHO. (2009b). *Road Traffic Injuries Publications and Resources: Related Resolutions*. Geneva: World Health Organization.

WHO. (2011). *Saving Millions of Lives: Decade of Action for Road Safety 2011–2020*. Geneva: World Health Organization.

WHO. (2015). *Global Status Report on Road Safety 2015*. Retrieved from Geneva: World Health Organization.

WHO. (2016). *Addressing the Challenges of the United Nations Decade of Action for Road Safety (2011–2020): Outcome of the Second Global High-level Conference on Road Safety: Time for Results*. Geneva: WHO. http://apps.who.int/gb/ebwha/pdf_files/WHA69/A69_R7-en.pdf

WHO. (2018). *Global Status Report on Road Safety 2018 (9241565683)*. Retrieved from Geneva: WHO.

Williams, A. F., & O'Neill, B. (1974). On-the-road driving records of licensed race drivers. *Accident Analysis & Prevention, 6*(3–4), 263–270.

Zaouk, A., Willis, M., Traube, E., & Strassburger, R. (2015). Driver alcohol detection system for safety (DADSS): A non-regulatory approach in the development and deployment of vehicle safety technology to reduce alcohol-impaired driving: A status update. 24th International Technical Conference on the Enhanced Safety of Vehicles (ESV), Gothenburg.

APPENDIX

Table A11.1: Country Codes: Two letter codes in the chart denote countries listed in the chapter

Code	Country/Area
AF	Afghanistan
BD	Bangladesh
BT	Bhutan
KH	Cambodia
CN	China
IN	India
ID	Indonesia
IR	Iran (Islamic Republic of)
JP	Japan
JO	Jordan
KW	Kuwait
LA	Lao People's Democratic Republic
MY	Malaysia
MV	Maldives
MM	Myanmar
NP	Nepal
OM	Oman
PK	Pakistan
PH	Philippines
QA	Qatar
KR	Republic of Korea
SA	Saudi Arabia
SG	Singapore
LK	Sri Lanka
TH	Thailand
AE	United Arab Emirates
VN	Viet Nam

SECTION III

HEALTH PROMOTION PRACTICES IN DIFFERENT SETTINGS

A Perspective: Health Promotion in a Complex World

Glenn Laverack

We live in a complex world in which problems cannot be resolved with simple perspectives and solutions. We need a bold vision for the future of health promotion to match the complexity of the 21st century. Health promotion must continue to evolve by making key decisions collectively and in an open and inclusive process of dialogue to ensure that the broader professional interests are represented and preserved. The challenges of the past remind us of the need for a vision based on robust multinational collaboration and strong individual leadership. We must invest in health promotion services, build professional and community capacities, and target the most vulnerable populations.[1] To stay ahead of emerging health trends and infectious diseases we must invest in surveillance, the behavioral and social sciences, and empowerment.

The single major cause of poor global health is poverty, underscored by social injustice and disempowerment. Poor health is a symptom of an inequitable society and this is why it is important to persevere integrating the social determinants into health promotion as a step toward dealing with the "causes of the causes". We are also faced with an enormous backlog of prevention, care, and treatment, a consequence of the coronavirus pandemic. This has been the worst health crisis for more than a century, impacting the lives, health, and well-being of billions of people worldwide.

The coronavirus pandemic has shown us how fragile the world is, how unprepared health services are, and how quickly democratic and economic systems can be disrupted.[2] Health promotion can play a crucial role during an infectious disease outbreak including the use of communication and bottom-up approaches to ensure that communities are engaged in a sustainable and positive way. This is an exciting new development for health promotion that must be equal to its role to address noncommunicable diseases.[3]

Other emerging priorities in a complex world include planetary health, digital transformation, universal health coverage, health literacy, and the commercial determinants of health. However, there are also a number of unresolved health promotion priorities including the transition from health education and individual responsibility to national health promotion models and building professional cultural competence. We must ensure that the priorities of the past are being resolved while moving forward with a new vision for health promotion in the 21st century.

There is an urgency to map out how health promotion can make a significant contribution to addressing the inequity, social injustice, and poverty in society. This does not require a major operational shift because many of its activities already enable people to increase control over their health and well-being and to influence the determinants of their health. Globally, it is essential for international organizations and professional bodies to work together to ensure that health promotion is unified in achieving poverty alleviation. In a complex world, health promotion has an important role to build healthier, more sustainable, and more equitable societies.

NOTES

1. EuroHealthNet (2021) Investing in health promotion services. Beyond the Health Sector – Financing e-Guide (health-inequalities.eu).

2. Kickbusch, I. (2021) Visioning the future of health promotion. *Global Health Promotion* 28(4): 56–63.

3. Laverack, G. (2018) *Health promotion in disease outbreaks and health emergencies.* Boca Raton, FL, CRC Press/Taylor & Francis Group.

 DOI: 10.1201/b23385-21

12 Health Promotion for Prevention and Control of Cancer in Low- and Middle-Income Countries

Krithiga Shridhar, Ravi Mehrotra, and Preet K. Dhillon

CONTENTS

> The function of protecting and developing health must rank even above that of restoring it when it is impaired.
>
> **Hippocrates**
>
> It is far easier and more effective to prevent cancer than to treat it.
>
> **World Health Organization**

KEY MESSAGES

- Cancer is a global public health priority, particularly affecting low- and middle-income countries (LMICs) more in terms of mortality, morbidity, low survival, and poor quality of life.
- The most disadvantaged groups in LMICs further suffer disproportionately from inequitable health care access and cancer illiteracy, leading to late diagnosis and poor prognosis.
- Leading cancer types are largely preventable and/or amenable to early detection and timely treatment, and a majority of other cancer types need appropriate and adequate treatment and palliation. Early detection and timely treatment are key elements to lowering morbidity due to cancer.
- Health promotion approaches could (1) control risk factors and promote vaccination for reducing cancer incidence (primary prevention); (2) increase uptake of screening, early detection, and timely treatment for reducing cancer mortality (secondary prevention); and (3) improve access to affordable treatment and palliation for a better quality of life and survival (tertiary care).
- Cancer prevention and control through universal health coverage efforts are critical for addressing the cancer burden and inequities in LMIC populations.
- Improving cancer literacy and reducing stigma are also important components of health promotion for cancer prevention and treatment in the continuity of cancer care.

INTRODUCTION

More than half of all cancers and two-thirds of cancer deaths occur in low- and middle-income countries (LMICs; 58.6% and 70% in 2018) (1). Cancer is the second leading cause of death globally, and in LMICs, patients with cancer have late diagnosis and poorer prognosis compared to high-income countries (HICs), due to the lack of or inequitable access to health services and inadequate cancer literacy. Lifestyle, environmental and occupational factors, and infections, as well as certain

DOI: 10.1201/b23385-22

host-level factors including genetic susceptibility are the known risk factors for cancer. Depending on the cancer type and prevalence of known modifiable risk factors in a population, nearly 40% of all cancers and more than 90% of certain specific cancers can be prevented by removing the most important carcinogenic exposures (2).

HEALTH PROMOTION APPROACHES FOR CANCER PREVENTION AND CONTROL

Well-planned health promotion activities enable cancer prevention and control at three levels: (1) primary prevention approaches to reduce risk exposures or to increase individuals' resistance to them through vaccination can lower cancer incidence; (2) secondary prevention approaches by screening, early detection, and timely treatment can prevent cancer progression and reduce mortality; and (3) tertiary care approaches for adequate treatment and rehabilitation can control cancer morbidity, improve quality of life and survivorship (Figure 12.1). The World Health Organization's (WHO) International Agency for Research on Cancer (IARC) provides evidence-based guidance on cancer prevention and control, which is implemented by individual countries through National Cancer Control Plans (https://www.iarc.fr/). Globally and in LMICs, the leading cancer types (Tables 12.1 and 12.2) are largely preventable and/or amenable to screening, early detection, and timely treatment.

CANCER PREVENTION EDUCATION AT SCHOOLS, INTERVENTIONS IN WORK SETTINGS, AND COMMUNITY ENGAGEMENT

Schools provide a good platform for the delivery of cancer-related knowledge for adolescents aged 13–19 years through lectures or peer-group teaching. In developing countries, there is a need to focus on the basic awareness of definitions, common risk factors, and symptoms across wide socio-economic, literacy, and urban–rural divides. In developed countries, these programs exist along with discussions on the benefits and risks of vaccinations, screening tests, and genetic testing to determine individualized risks. Cancer prevention interventions in *workplaces* to reach adults are effective in HICs (e.g., Gold Standard Accreditation programs in the US). These range from organizational policies to protect and minimize occupational exposures to carcinogens, facilitating smoke-free environments, serving healthy food, offering breastfeeding spaces, and promoting and providing on-site cancer screening and early detection for common cancers. This is more challenging in LMIC settings, but interventions at work settings for cancer prevention can be made sustainable by integrating them with workplace initiatives for other chronic conditions. In many LMIC settings, a large section is unorganized making it more challenging.

Community engagement is enhanced through the participation of nongovernmental organizations (NGOs), auxiliary health workers, patient advocacy groups, tertiary hospital initiatives, and media. The American Cancer Society, Union for International Cancer Control, and Cancer

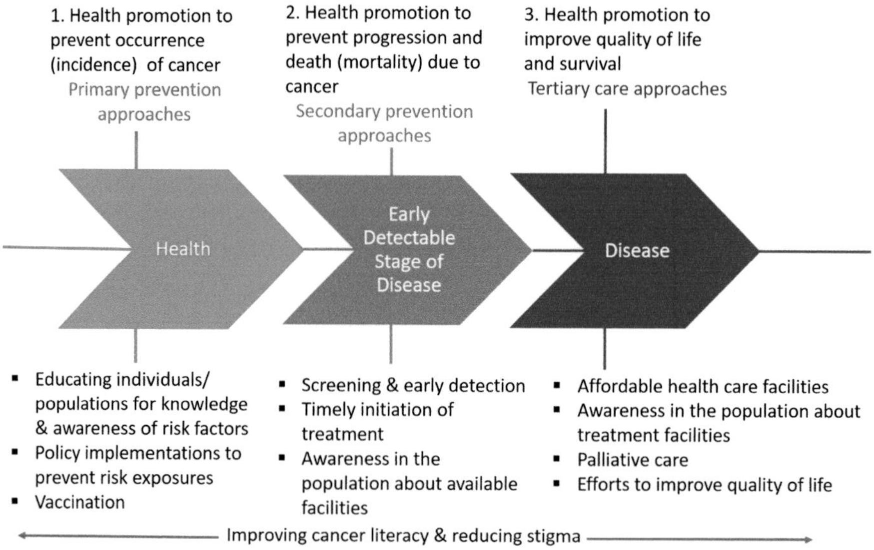

Figure 12.1 Health promotion for cancer prevention and control.

Table 12.1: Top Five Cancer Sites in Men Based on Incidence

Cancer Site	Incidence (ASR/100,000)	Mortality (ASR/100,000)
Global		
Lung	31.5	27.1
Prostate	29.3	7.6
Colorectum	23.6	10.8
Stomach	15.7	11.7
Liver	13.9	12.7
All sites	218.6	122.7
HICs		
Prostate	64.1	8.6
Lung	39.1	29.0
Colorectum	37.3	13.3
Bladder	18.6	4.2
Stomach	14.5	6.3
All sites	341.8	118.6
LMICs		
Lung	28.2	25.9
Colorectum	18.2	9.7
Prostate	16.7	7.0
Stomach	16.0	13.7
Liver	14.8	14.0
All sites	171.2	120.9

Sources: GLOBOCAN 2018; https://gco.iarc.fr/today/.

Table 12.2: Top Five Cancer Sites in Women Based on Incidence

Cancer Site	Incidence (ASR/100,000)	Mortality (ASR/100,000)
Global		
Breast	46.3	13.0
Colorectum	16.3	7.2
Lung	14.6	11.2
Cervix	13.1	6.9
Thyroid	10.2	0.4
All sites	182.6	83.1
HIC		
Breast	78.3	12.9
Colorectum	25.1	8.4
Lung	23.1	15.0
Thyroid	9.8	0.35
Corpus uteri	15.5	2.4
All sites	278.0	79.5
LMICs		
Breast	36.5	12.8
Cervix	14.5	8.2
Colorectum	14.4	6.6
Lung	12.7	9.7
Thyroid	8.7	0.53
All sites	151.0	82.3

Sources: GLOBOCAN 2018; https://gco.iarc.fr/today/.

Council Australia in HICs; and Malaysian cancer NGOs and the Chinese Anti-Cancer Association in LMICs are a few good examples. In India, NGOs such as the Indian Cancer Society and Cancer Foundation of India are key contributors to cancer prevention and control. Their activities include creating awareness of risk factors and the importance of regular check-ups, conducting screening camps, providing information on treatment and rehabilitation, supporting patient navigation, and facilitating psychosocial and financial support. NGOs can be trained to manage population-based cancer registries such as the Indian Cancer Society in the cities of Maharashtra Mumbai, Pune, Nagpur, and Aurangabad in India. NGOs also play a crucial role in affordable cancer treatment in India. Reputable tertiary care centers – Cancer Institutes at Chennai, Nagpur, Gwalior, and Ahmedabad – are operated through NGOs.

BOX 12.1 WORKSITE AND COMMUNITY INTERVENTIONS IN LMICS

In Uganda, where cervical cancer screening uptake is low due to limited access, a community self-collected human papillomavirus (HPV) testing and treatment for women is found to be effective. Trials to integrate it with an existing national health program are underway. An attempt with mobile health and task-sharing enabled cost-effective specialist care for oral cancer screening and early detection in rural Indian settings. Trained health workers screened individuals door-to-door and in workplaces and followed up with specialists remotely for continuum care.

POLICY IMPLEMENTATIONS FOR REDUCTION OF RISK FACTORS

(a) Tobacco, betel quid, and harmful use of alcohol are the major preventable risk factors associated with cancers. The WHO's MPOWER measures for tobacco control and its Framework Convention on Tobacco Control (WHO FCTC, 2003) benefit over 5 billion people worldwide, out of which about two-thirds reside in LMICs. This includes taxing products, bans on advertising and marketing, health warnings, monitoring tobacco control policies, and providing support for habit cessation. These measures often need modifications in the regional context. Policy restrictions for smokeless tobacco as well as betel quid and areca nut, globally and in LMICs, are still inadequate. Currently, no global policy exists for the control of smokeless tobacco, nevertheless, the WHO MPOWER FCTC can provide a template for future action. In contrast to tobacco, alcohol restriction policies are hampered by disagreements about problem definition (heavy vs. regular vs. episodic binge drinking) and proper focus of policy solutions (licensing system, drunk driving, alcohol dependency, and recovery). The situation is complex in LMICs where the level of awareness is low among the populations and policymakers.

(b) Diet and physical activity recommendations include (3):

- Maintain a healthy weight and be physically active.
- Eat a diet rich in whole grains, vegetables, fruits, and beans.
- Limit consumption of processed red meat, fast foods, and processed foods high in fat or sugars.
- Do not use supplements for cancer prevention.
- Mothers should breastfeed their babies.

The larger perspective of diet and physical activity stems from national-level policies. The local food environment controls the decision to eat fruits, vegetables, pulses, and fish versus processed and ready-to-eat food items, and the availability of meat. A household in a low-resource setting, such as India, on average spends approximately 50% of its monthly income on five servings of fruits and vegetables/day/person (vs. <2% in HICs). On the contrary, in HICs, where resources, knowledge, and awareness complement one another, the implementation of necessary policies can translate into immediate benefits.

(c) *Occupational and environmental exposure* to asbestos, wood/leather/rubber/paint dust, coal tar, silica, heavy metals (lead, arsenic, chromium, cadmium), toxic chemicals (pesticides), engine/diesel exhaust, fumes and smoke, outdoor (PM2.5) and indoor air, water and soil pollution, and radiation are established human carcinogens linked to cancers of the aerodigestive tract, skin, and blood (4). Key drivers of these types of pollution are uncontrolled urbanization and industrialization with deforestation and increasing use of toxic chemicals. Globally, in 2015, 40% of lung cancer deaths were attributed to occupational and environmental air pollution, gases, and fumes, and the proportional lung cancer disabilities attributable to tobacco and pollution were almost equal, disproportionately affecting LMICs (4). Household air pollution by the burning of coal and solid fuels also remains a major concern in the majority of these settings for increasing lung cancers among women. Latin America, the Caribbean, and certain Asian countries including China have recently implemented intersectoral plans for control of air, water, and soil pollution (4). India enacted the National Clean Air Programme in 2019. Occupational and environmental health needs intersectoral efforts ranging from awareness and knowledge, and social mobilization to effective policy recommendations and impact evaluation.

VACCINATIONS

Vaccinations to prevent cervical and liver cancers are one of the "best buy" interventions of the WHO for LMICs. Chronic infection with hepatitis B virus (HBV) is one of the most important causes of liver cancer, and highly effective vaccines have been available since 1982. Taiwan and China were the countries to first offer the HBV vaccine, resulting in a marked decrease in liver cancers. By 2016, 185 countries had introduced HBV vaccination as routine childhood immunization, with 87% coverage globally. Cervical cancers can be prevented through HPV vaccination. Broad implementation of HPV vaccination began at the end of 2006, initially in developed countries such as the United States, Canada, Australia, and United Kingdom. High coverage has generally been achieved, due to school-based vaccination programs and the promotion of routine coadministration of HPV vaccines with standard vaccines. Low-income countries in Asia and Africa, including Rwanda, Bhutan, Ghana, Kenya, Lao, Madagascar, Malawi, Niger, Sierra Leone, and Tanzania, where the burden of cervical cancer was high, implemented HPV vaccines either in national schedule or as demonstration projects (5). Unlike HBV vaccines, relatively high costs, a protracted timeframe for administration (adolescent girls), and antivaccination campaigns hamper universal coverage of HPV immunization.

BOX 12.2 IMPACT OF HPV VACCINATIONS AND CHALLENGES IN LMICS

Australia, the first country to implement HPV vaccination in school-based programs, reported a significant decrease in high-grade precancerous cervical lesions in girls aged 15–19 years old. There are only three countries in the South Asian region that have implemented the HPV vaccination: Thailand, Malaysia, and Laos. Whereas Thailand and Malaysia are upper-middle-income countries, Laos is a lower-middle-income country and the sustainability of the program is a challenge. In Thailand, the market price has considerably come down since 2010, making the program more sustainable. In Malaysia, HPV vaccines have been provided for free since 2010 for girls and women up to age 26 at any of the government clinics nationwide, and the vaccine coverage in 2011 was 87%. Both Thailand and Malaysia have successfully maintained vaccine coverage among their target population. Data from Indian states such as Punjab, which has implemented a school-based HPV vaccination program (class 6 girls); Delhi, which has initiated free HPV vaccination through Delhi State Cancer Institutes for girls aged 11–13 years; and Sikkim, which offers routine immunization for girls 9–13 years, can help scale-up implementation.

From https://www.who.int/ncds/surveillance/data-toolkit-for-cervical-cancer-prevention-control/en/

SCREENING AND EARLY DETECTION FOR SECONDARY PREVENTION

Screening is applied to a defined population to identify asymptomatic disease using simple tests, which are later confirmed using imaging, histology, and other diagnostic tests. Screening leads to earlier detection of cancers, some in a curable stage, and in general, leads to downstaging, as the prevalent disease is detected either asymptomatically or in symptomatic, earlier stages of the disease.

Organized screening at the population level requires (1) a cancer type of public health importance (high incidence and lethality in productive years) that can be either detected in the precancer stage (e.g., cervical, colorectal, oral cancers) or early cancer stage (e.g., breast cancer) and treated with a favorable outcome; (2) a reliable and valid screening test; and (3) a screening program linked to diagnostic and treatment facilities. Multiple challenges, including trained human resources, referral pathways, and cost-effectiveness as well as awareness about available facilities in the general population need to be addressed for the effective implementation of any screening program. However, not all cancers are amenable to screening and early detection, and a different health promotion approach may be considered (Box 12.3).

BOX 12.3 POTENTIAL HEALTH PROMOTION STRATEGIES FOR DIFFERENT CANCER TYPES

CANCERS PREVENTABLE BY RISK EXPOSURE REDUCTION

- Tobacco and alcohol: cancers of the head and neck, bladder, liver, lung, pancreas, esophagus
- Diet and physical activity: cancers of the stomach, colorectum, esophagus, breast, pancreas, endometrium
- Air pollution (indoor and outdoor): cancers of the lung, esophagus
- Human papillomavirus infection: cancers of the cervix (over 90%), head, and neck, particularly oropharyngeal cancers
- Hepatitis infection: hepatocellular (liver) cancer
- *H. pylori* infection (through hygienic living conditions): stomach cancer

CANCERS AMENABLE TO SCREENING, EARLY DETECTION, AND TIMELY TREATMENT

- Cervical cancer
- Breast cancer
- Colorectal cancer
- Oral cancer

CANCERS THAT ARE POTENTIALLY CURABLE WITH SYSTEMIC TREATMENT, FOR WHICH EARLY DETECTION IS LIMITED AND NOT CRITICAL

- Burkitt's lymphoma
- Large-cell lymphoma
- Hodgkin's lymphoma
- Testicular cancer
- Acute lymphoblastic leukemia
- Soft tissue sarcoma
- Osteosarcoma

CANCERS THAT ARE MANAGED THROUGH PALLIATIVE CARE*

- Kaposi's sarcoma
- Advanced breast cancer
- Ovarian cancer
- Chronic myelogenous leukemia

Adapted from Farmer P, Frenk J, Knaul FM, Shulman LN, Alleyne G, Armstrong L, et al., Expansion of cancer care and control in countries of low and middle income: A call to action, The Lancet, 2010;376(9747):1186–93; Sankaranarayanan R, Boffetta P, Research on cancer prevention, detection and management in low- and medium-income countries, Ann Oncol. 2010;21(10):1935–43; and World Cancer Report 2020, https://www.iarc.fr/cards_page/world-cancer-report/.

**"Palliative care is an approach that improves the quality of life of patients and their families facing the problem associated with life-threatening illness, through the prevention and relief of suffering using early identification and impeccable assessment and treatment of pain and other problems, physical, psychosocial and spiritual" (https://www.who.int/cancer/palliative/definition/en/).*

Note: For certain cancer types where the risk factors are not fully understood (gallbladder, kidney, brain, and thyroid cancers) and/or not generally modifiable (prostate cancer), and where early detection is less feasible (gallbladder cancer) or not recommended (prostate, thyroid, and kidney cancers) with an uncertain prognosis, health promotion strategies are currently limited, warranting rigorous epidemiological research.

BOX 12.4 CANCER SCREENING IN LMICS

Among LMICs, Sri Lanka, Mexico, and Thailand, with universal health care, offer free opportunistic cancer screenings and treatments at government facilities with equitable access to underserved populations (6). In India, population-based screenings of common cancers are being rolled out in phases for 30- to 65-year-old women for breast and cervix cancer, and for 30- to 65-year-old men and women (tobacco, betel quid, and alcohol users) for oral cancers. Clinical breast exams, visual exams with acetic acid for cervix cancer, and clinical exams for oral cancers are recommended, based on utility for downstaging and cost-effectiveness (Figure 12.2). Telementoring of primary healthcare providers through the Extension for Community Healthcare Outcomes program is initiated by the National Institute of Cancer Prevention and Research to train more human resources.

Type of Cancer	Age of beneficiary	Method of Screening	Frequency of screening	If positive
Oral	30 -65 years	Oral Visual Examination (OVE)	Once in 5years	Referred to Surgeon/Dentist/ENT specialist/Medical officer at CHC/ DH for confirmation* and biopsy.
Cervical	30-65 years	Visual Inspection with Acetic acid (VIA)	Once in 5years	Referred to the PHC/CHC/DH for further evaluation and management of pre-cancerous conditions where gynecologist/trained Lady Medical Officer is available.
Breast	30-65 years	Clinical Breast Examination (CBE)	Once in 5years	Referred to Surgeon at CHC/DH for confirmation using a Breast ultra sound probe followed by biopsy as appropriate.

*The biopsy specimen either to be sent to the nearest Medical college or using the mechanism under the Free Diagnostics Initiative under NHM,to the nearest NABL certified laboratory.

Figure 12.2 National cancer screening program framework in India. (From Operational Framework: Management of Common Cancers, p. 7, http://nicpr.in.)

HEALTH PROMOTION FOR TREATMENT, PALLIATIVE CARE, AND SURVIVORSHIP FOR TERTIARY PREVENTION

The inequalities in cancer survival rates across countries, particularly the low survival in LMICs, can be attributed to the unavailability of affordable and accessible quality healthcare facilities (7). The Global Task Force on Expanded Access to Cancer Care and Control in Developing Countries (GTF.CCC, 2009) initiates financing and procurement of affordable cancer drugs, vaccines, and treatment services. GTF.CCC works with the International Agency on Cancer Control, WHO, International Union Against Cancer, and other academic institutions and alliances in developed and developing countries (7). Successful programs such as treatment of multidrug-resistant tuberculosis and AIDS show that effective diagnosis and treatment can be introduced even in rural areas of low-income countries despite limited specialized services.

BOX 12.5 CIRCUMVENTING TREATMENT CHALLENGES IN LMICS: CASE STUDIES FROM DIFFERENT COUNTRIES

To counter limited healthcare access and specialized resources, an international partnership in rural Malawi, Rwanda, and Haiti trained local physicians and nurse teams to deliver chemotherapy to cancer patients (7).

Several Asian and Latin American countries are implementing large-scale insurance programs focusing on economically vulnerable sections of society. Mexico's Seguro Popular Catastrophic Insurance Fund and India's Ayushman Bharat Yojana are good examples.

A sustained supply of low-cost generic drugs is a critical step for improving access to essential medicines for cancer care in LMICs. For example, lenalidomide is an essential drug for treating multiple myeloma. In India, where it is not patent-protected, generic versions of the medicine are available at low cost, while in South Africa it is not (8).

In India, the National Cancer Grid was formed as a union of cancer centers, research institutes, patient groups, and charitable institutions in the country to provide evidence-based, uniform, and high-quality cancer care to all patients.

Community-based and home-based preventive health interventions may accelerate the improved quality of life for cancer survivors at risk of losing physical independence. Patient support groups associated with NGOs help to enhance peer support, which impacts positively not only on survivorship but also on the quality of life of people affected with cancer.

IMPROVING CANCER LITERACY AND REDUCING CANCER STIGMA

Increasing knowledge and awareness and reducing fear and stigma are effective strategies that impact health promotion along the cancer continuum. Contextually specific and culturally appropriate measures, and programs specifically for women (e.g., Breast Health Global Initiative) and socioeconomically disadvantaged groups are needed to address the challenges. "Community-pull" strategies, such as increasing literacy through rigorous dissemination of information through multiple stakeholders and national surveys and addressing psychosocial factors for stigma, are recommended for the effective implementation of cancer prevention and control programs in LMICs (9).

ROLE OF CANCER REGISTRIES

Cancer registries are surveillance systems that help us understand the burden and distribution of disease and identify risk factors for prevention and control in a geographically defined population.

Statistics on the occurrence of cancer in population-based cancer registry reports provide the necessary framework to:

1. Monitor the burden of disease in terms of incidence, mortality, trends, and survival.
2. Investigate new exposures in terms of etiological research and their prevention.
3. Plan health delivery systems for cancer control activities in populations.

SUMMARY

The United Nations' 2030 Agenda for Sustainable Development highlights cancer as a major public health priority for governments across the globe. In LMICs, cancer is one of the important contributors to health loss due to late-stage diagnosis and poor survival. Health promotion could improve cancer prevention and control at three levels, including control of risk factors and vaccination; increasing uptake of screening, early detection, and timely treatment; and improving access to affordable tertiary care for treatment and palliation care for a better quality of life in cancer survivorship. Improving cancer literacy and reducing stigma further impact health promotion activities at each of these levels. Cancer registries are a unique resource that can be harnessed to enable or stimulate these activities. LMICs face challenges in generating culturally appropriate messages and context-specific awareness programs on risk factors, implementation of screening programs, resource distribution for treatment and palliation, developing appropriate policies, and discussing genetic susceptibility. Effective cancer health promotion activities are better translated through universal health coverage efforts. This is critical for addressing the cancer burden and inequities in LMIC populations, which disproportionately fall upon their rural, migrant, women, elderly, poor, and less educated populations. The context of limited tertiary care facilities for cancer care makes access to cancer treatments difficult for the poor.

REFERENCES

1. Ferlay J, Ervik M, Lam F, Colombet M, Mery L, Piñeros M, et al. Global cancer observatory: Cancer today. Lyon, France: International Agency for Research on Cancer. Available from: https://gco.iarc.fr/today, accessed [20-06-2020]. 2018.

2. Bray F, Soerjomataram I. Population attributable fractions continue to unmask the power of prevention. *Br J Cancer.* 2018;118(8):1031–2.

3. World Cancer Research Fund International. *Diet, Nutrition, Physical Activity and Cancer: A Global Perspective.* 2018. Available from: Cancer Prevention Organisation | World Cancer Research Fund International, accessed [20-06-2020]. 2018.

4. Landrigan PJ, Fuller R, Acosta NJR, Adeyi O, Arnold R, Basu NN, et al. The Lancet Commission on Pollution and Health. *Lancet.* 2018;391(10119):462–512.

5. El-Zein M, Richardson L, Franco EL. Cervical cancer screening of HPV vaccinated populations: Cytology, molecular testing, both or none. *Journal of Clinical Virology: The Official Publication of the Pan American Society for Clinical Virology.* 2016;76(Suppl 1):S62–S8.

6. Sivaram S, Majumdar G, Perin D, Nessa A, Broeders M, Lynge E, et al. Population-based cancer screening programmes in low-income and middle-income countries: Regional consultation of the International Cancer Screening Network in India. *Lancet Oncol.* 2018;19(2): e113–e22.

7. Farmer P, Frenk J, Knaul FM, Shulman LN, Alleyne G, Armstrong L, et al. Expansion of cancer care and control in countries of low and middle income: A call to action. *Lancet.* 2010;376(9747):1186–93.

8. 't Hoen E, Meyer S, Durisch P, Bannenberg W, Perehudoff K, Reed T, et al. Improving affordability of new essential cancer medicines. *The Lancet Oncology.* 2019 Aug 1;20(8):1052–4.

9. Krishnan S, Sivaram S, Anderson BO, Basu P, Belinson JL, Bhatla N, et al. Using implementation science to advance cancer prevention in India. *Asian Pacific Journal of Cancer Prevention: APJCP.* 2015;16(9):3639–44.

SUGGESTED READING

World Cancer Report 2020. World Health Organization and International Agency for Research on Cancer; 2020. Lyon (France). Available at https://www.iarc.fr/cards_page/world-cancer-report/

Textbook: Cancer Epidemiology: Principles and Methods. dos Santos Silva I, editor: World Health Organization and International Agency for Research on Cancer; 1999. Lyon (France).

Acknowledgments

We are thankful to Eliza Dutta, a post-doctoral researcher at the Public Health Foundation of India, for editing and formatting.

13 Health Promotion Is Site-Specific

Muralidhar M. Kulkarni, Ranjitha S. Shetty, and Chythra R. Rao

CONTENTS

> It is health that is the real wealth and not the pieces of gold and silver.
>
> **Mahatma Gandhi**

INTRODUCTION

Health promotion is the process of enabling people to increase control over and improve their health in order to reach a state of complete physical, mental, and social well-being, and change or cope with the environment.[1]

According to the World Health Organization (WHO), the five implementing strategies for health promotion are building healthy public policy, creating supportive environments, strengthening community actions, developing personal skills, and reorienting health services as elaborated in the Ottawa Charter.[2,3]

These strategies and programs should be adapted to the local needs taking into account the differing social, cultural, and economic systems of individual countries and regions.[3]

In the current health scenario wherein the world is facing a 'triple burden of disease' – constituted by the unfinished agenda of communicable diseases, unprecedented rise of chronic noncommunicable diseases, as well as the health issues caused by climate change – the principles of health promotion need to be strengthened with simple, cost-effective, innovative, and culturally and geographically appropriate models holistically embedded with other forms of healthcare to ensure better population health.[4]

As emphasized in the Ottawa Charter in the year 1986, "Health is created and lived by people within the settings of their everyday life; where they learn, work, play, and love." Settings can be identified as having physical boundaries, a range of people with defined roles, and an organizational structure in which people engage in daily activities wherein environmental, organizational, and personal factors interact to affect health and well-being. These settings can also be used to promote health, as they are vehicles to reach individuals, gain access to services, and synergistically bring together favorable interactions.[1,5] The important influence of the environmental context on health, which includes place, setting, and multiple environments, has directed health promotion practitioners to focus on changing settings for the promotion of individual and community health instead of targeting individuals.[6] Some common examples of settings are depicted in Figure 13.1.[8]

HEALTH PROMOTION IN SCHOOL SETTINGS

Health promotion in a school setting could be defined as any activity undertaken to improve and/or protect the health of all school users. It is a broader concept than health education, and it includes provision and activities relating to healthy school policies, the school's physical and social environment, integrated health curriculum, community links, and health services as shown in Figure 13.2.[9]

DOI: 10.1201/b23385-23

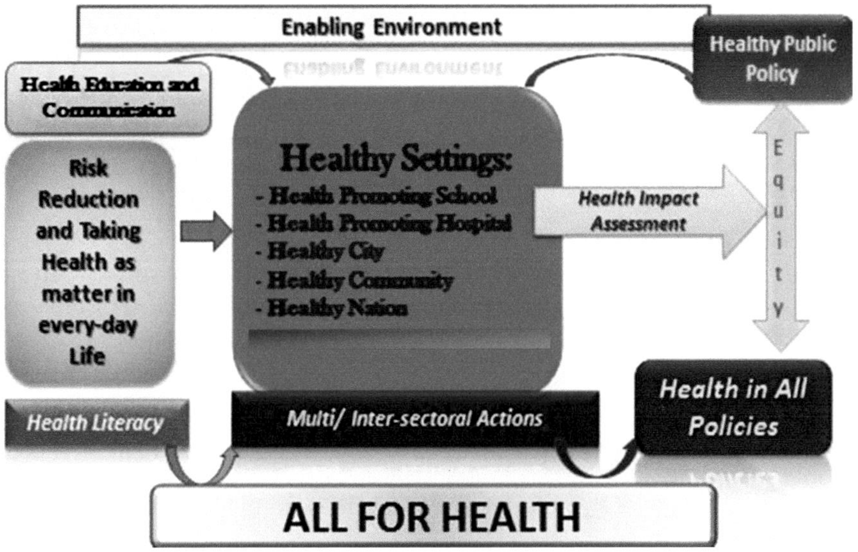

Figure 13.1 Framework for health promotion actions.[7]

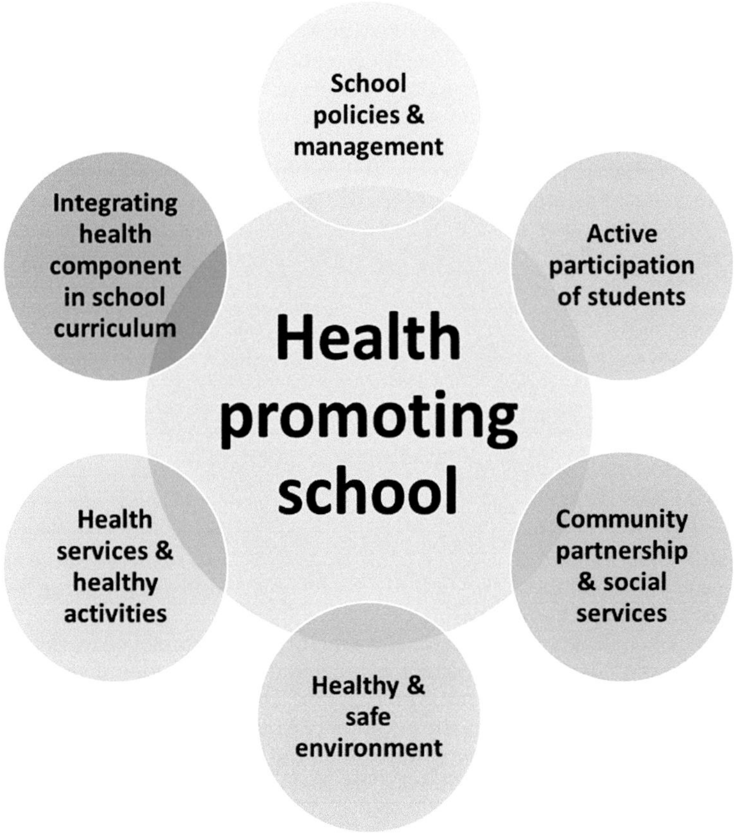
School policies & management
Integrating health component in school curriculum
Active participation of students
Health promoting school
Health services & healthy activities
Community partnership & social services
Healthy & safe environment

Figure 13.2 Components of a health promoting school.

A health-promoting school constantly strengthens its capacity as a healthy setting for living, learning, and working. The WHO describes it as one that fosters health and learning with all measures at its disposal and engages health and education officials, teachers, students, and parents in the efforts to make the school a healthy place.[10,11]

Worldwide, education and health are inextricably linked. Healthy young people are more likely to learn more effectively. Health promotion can assist schools to meet their targets in educational attainment and social aims. Young people who feel good about their school and who are connected to significant adults are less likely to undertake high-risk behaviors and are likely to have better learning outcomes.[9]

Strategies for Health Promotion in Schools

Whole-School Approach (Health Promoting School Policies and Environment)

A Cochrane Review reported strong evidence to support the beneficial effects of child obesity prevention programs on body mass index (BMI), particularly for programs targeted at children aged 6 to 12 years.[12]

Langford et al. provided evidence that education and health are interrelated. The Cochrane analysis of the health promoting schools framework showed effectiveness in interventions like a reduction in students' BMI, changes in physical activity, improvement in intake of fruits and vegetables, reduction in the use of cigarettes, and reduced incidents of being bullied.[13]

mHealth Initiatives

'SWAP IT' assessed the potential efficacy, feasibility, and acceptability of an mhealth intervention to improve the energy and nutritional quality of foods packed in children's lunchboxes. A large proportion (71%) of parents reported awareness of the intervention, making healthier swaps in lunchboxes (55%), and pushed content was helpful (84%).[14]

Multicomponent Intervention

The multicomponent whole-school SEHER health promotion intervention in grade 9 students (aged 13–14 years) at government-run secondary schools in the Nalanda district of Bihar state, India, had substantial beneficial effects on school climate and health-related outcomes when delivered by lay counselors.[15]

Project MYTRI (Mobilizing Youth for Tobacco-Related Initiatives) was a multicomponent intervention comprising behavioral classroom curricula, school posters, a parental involvement component, and peer-led activism intended to prevent tobacco use among Indian adolescents. It demonstrated that the overall tobacco use among school-going adolescents decreased by 17% after intervention, while it increased by 68% in the control group.[16]

Life Course Approach

A life course approach focusing on the school-going age groups involving policy, advocacy, and legislation; the food and beverage industry; the media; and the built environment can provide opportunities for children and adolescents to make healthy choices and provide opportunities for safe physical activity beginning early in life.[17]

HEALTH PROMOTION IN WORKPLACES

In India, the workforce has been increasing substantially due to rapid industrialization and a growing economy.[18,19] Workplaces offer easy and regular access to a relatively large and stable population at a time with sustained peer support and an opportunity to influence behavior at individual and organizational levels.[18,20]

Evidence shows that employee health status directly influences employee work behavior, work attendance, and on-the-job performance, which is reiterated by international agencies such as the WHO and International Labor Organization (ILO).[21,22] The WHO's Global Plan of Action on Worker's Health 2008–2017 also endorses the point that health promotion and prevention of noncommunicable diseases should be further stimulated in the workplace.[18] Enhanced physical activity, breaking of uninterrupted sitting, healthier diets, and prohibition of tobacco use are amenable to be addressed at workplaces.

Evidence for Effectiveness of Health Promotion in Workplaces

There is extensive evidence on the role of workplace interventions in making employees healthier. A systematic review and meta-analysis assessed the effects of educational/behavioral interventions, environmental modifications, and multicomponent interventional strategies in workplaces on reducing sedentary time among white-collar workers. The review concluded that providing alternative workstations, treadmill workstations, and promoting stair use for the employees had positive outcomes.[23]

Similarly, interventions such as having educational workshops/campaigns, wellness fairs, disseminating information through brochures/internet, and incentivizing employees on achieving goals have been found to be effective in improving the cardiometabolic health of working adults.[24]

BOX 13.1

A multicentric study was carried out among employees of ten industries across different regions of India. The study adopted multicomponent intervention strategies comprised of sessions with individual employees and their families, displaying motivational tips on banners and posters fixed at strategic locations in the workplaces, periodically providing handouts and booklets, and showing educational videos on health promotion. The study reported a significant reduction in the proportion of individuals with a Framingham ten-year risk score of ≥10% in the intervention groups (from 34.1% at baseline to 26.8%) as compared to control groups.[29]

In the process of planning and implementing workplace health promotion (WHP) programs, it is essential to identify the characteristics of best practices.[18] Important characteristics of a WHP program that would increase the participation level are having a multicomponent intervention to offer choices for a variety of participants, provision of monetary incentives/gift vouchers upon successful completion of the program, and devising a program that demands minimal time commitment with a targeted approach.[25,26] Linking the program to the organization's corporate objectives is another important feature of a successful WHP. This would enable employees to enjoy better health and life satisfaction, while it also supports employers by avoiding unnecessary health costs, reducing absenteeism, and enhancing productivity.[18] This strategy would also ensure the sustainability of the WHP program. The crucial barriers to making a WHP program a success in many of the sites included time constraints during working hours, lack of interest among the employees toward adapting lifestyle interventions, and working in shifts.[25,27]

The process of developing a WHP program would start with identifying peoples' needs, values, and priority issues that would help in mobilizing them to invest in change. This will be followed by assembling a health workforce team to bring about change in the workplace. This team would assess the baseline data on workplace conditions, workers' health, and the desired future of the work community. Following this, issues directly related to health such as preventing exposure to occupational hazards and those changes that would yield quick benefits need to be prioritized. Based on the priorities, a health plan should be devised, implemented, and periodically evaluated (Figure 13.3). The whole WHP revolves around two core principles: employer and employee involvement.[22]

To summarize, various interventional studies of WHP have shown promising outcomes, and these interventions have also been found to be cost-effective in many settings.[28] Periodic evaluation of the implemented WHP program should be incorporated on a regular basis, leading to its effective implementation with favorable outcomes.[29]

HEALTH PROMOTION IN COMMUNITY SETTINGS

A healthy city or community aims to create a health-supportive environment, achieve a good quality of life, provide basic sanitation and hygiene needs, and support access to healthcare. Being a healthy community depends not only on the existing health infrastructure, but also upon a commitment to improve a city's environs and a willingness to forge the necessary connections in political, economic, and social arenas to fulfill the aforementioned aims.[30,31]

The Shanghai consensus on healthy cities puts forth five governance principles for ensuring healthy cities: integrating health as a core consideration in all policies; addressing all determinants of health including social, environmental, and economic aspects; promoting strong community engagement; reorienting health and social services toward equity; and assessing and monitoring well-being, disease burden, and health determinants.[32]

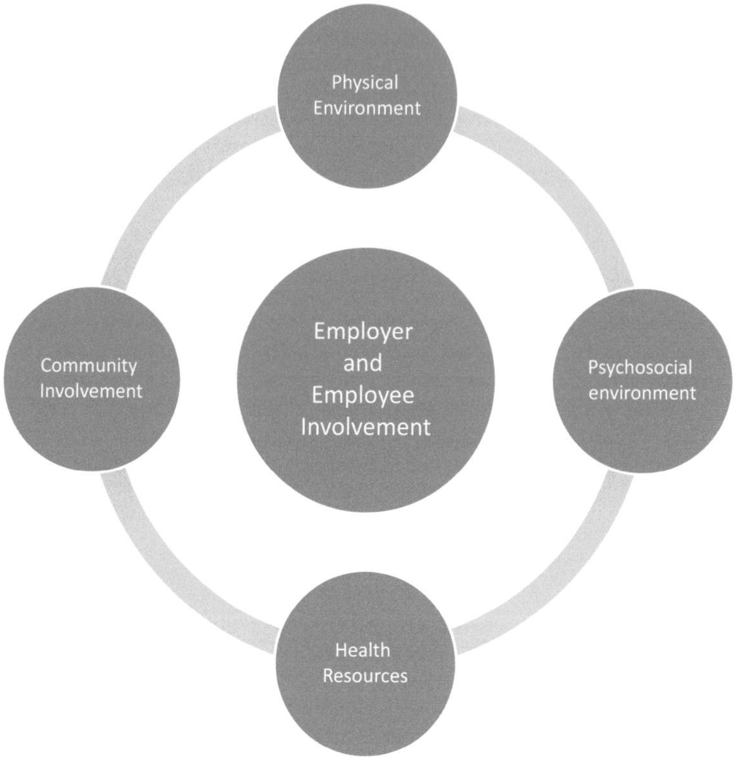

Figure 13.3 Healthy workplace model. (Adapted from the WHO healthy workplace model.)

The Government of India, under the National Health Mission, has initiated the formation of a village health and sanitation committee to provide a number of health and nutrition services and counseling to the community on a predesignated day, time, and place. Every month on a designated day the grassroots workers of the Department of Health and Family Welfare and the Department of Women and Child Development are responsible for mobilizing the community, with support from Panchayati Raj institutions, and holding health education sessions.[33,34] The presence of all these frontline workers is critical for the provision of the intended package of services. This strategy serves as an example that could be emulated elsewhere for health promotion in the community.

HEALTH PROMOTION IN HEALTHCARE SETTINGS

The importance of a well-functioning health system is emphasized by the WHO for achieving universal health promotion. The health system comprising of the health workforce and institutions should be well-financed, have universal reach, adequate manpower, mechanisms for community participation, and strong leadership in order to efficiently deliver comprehensive care.[1] Strengthening health systems is therefore a key strategy and priority for health promotion.

The recent National Health Policy 2017 in India recognizes and builds upon preventive and promotive care. The policy lays greater emphasis on investment and action in school, workplace, community, and healthcare settings with a focus on disease prevention and health promotion.[35]

In February 2018, the Government of India announced transforming existing sub health centers and primary health centers under the Ayushman Bharat Scheme. Ayushman Bharath's first component commits to strengthening the existing sub and primary health centers as health and wellness centers. The health-seeking behavior can be substantially improved if these centers are empowered to provide primary care concerning health promotion and disease prevention under one umbrella.[36] This lays the foundation for health promotion through a process of population empanelment, regular home and community interactions, and people's participation.[36] It aims to provide preventive, promotive, rehabilitative, and curative care for an expanded range of services encompassing reproductive and child health services, communicable diseases, noncommunicable diseases, palliative care and elderly care, oral health, and basic emergency care. The not-for-profit agencies and private sectors including medical schools have an opportunity to join with the government to strengthen healthcare services at the grassroots level under the public–private partnership model.[36] This is likely to further strengthen healthcare settings and contribute toward health promotion in the population.

Besides the primary care centers, there is ample opportunity for strengthening health promotion at hospitals that are predominantly focusing on curative and rehabilitative services. One of the key strategies identified in the Ottawa Charter was the reorientation of health services. Hospitals provide considerable opportunities to engage a broad section of the community through patients and their family members as well as their staff and personnel.[1] The WHO Regional Office for Europe started the first international consultations in 1988, followed by the European Pilot Hospital Project in 1993 in 20 partner hospitals in 11 European countries. The European Pilot Hospital Project focuses on four areas, namely, promoting the health of patients, promoting the health of staff, changing the organization to a health promoting setting, and promoting the health of the community in the catchment area of the hospital.[37]

The International Network of Health Promoting Hospitals (HPH) acts as a network linking all national/regional networks. In total, it consists of 38 national/regional HPH networks, collaborating to reorient healthcare toward the active promotion of health, with 800 hospital and health service members in more than 40 countries.[38]

CONCLUSION

Health is multifactorial with many factors from within the scope of the health system. The current scenario of epidemiologic and demographic transition, climate change, industrialization, migration, and global warming has exerted a tremendous negative impact on human health. In these circumstances, health promotion through a settings approach can positively modify the current challenges and lead to better health for the populace. As highlighted, there is a need and scope to provide supportive environments for health promotion in all settings in order to facilitate children and adults adopting appropriate measures that can go a long way in building a healthier society.

REFERENCES

1. World Health Organization (WHO). Website of the global conferences on health promotion. [Internet]. [cited 2020 Sep 27]. Available from: https://www.who.int/healthpromotion/conferences/en/
2. Lee CY, Kim HS, Ahn YH, Ko IS, Cho YH. Development of a community health promotion center based on the World Health Organization's Ottawa charter health promotion strategies. *Japan J Nurs Sci.* 2009;6(2):83–90.
3. Fortune K, Becerra-Posada F, Buss P, Galvão LAC, Contreras A, Murphy M, et al. Health promotion and the agenda for sustainable development, WHO region of the Americas. *Bull World Health Organ.* 2018;96(9):621–6.
4. Kumar S, Preetha GS. Health promotion: An effective tool for global health. *Indian J Community Med.* 2012;37(1):5–12.
5. Krech R. Healthy public policies: Looking ahead. *Health Promot Int.* 2011;26(SUPPL. 2):268–72.
6. Sallis JF, Cervero RB, Ascher W, Henderson KA, Kraft MK, Kerr J. An ecological approach to creating active living communities. *Ann Rev Public Health.* 2006;27:297–322.
7. World Health Organization (WHO). Framework for health promotion actions [Internet]. [cited 2020 Oct 12]. Available from: http://origin.searo.who.int/entity/healthpromotion/health-promotion-strategies/en/
8. World Health Organization (WHO). Healthy settings [Internet]. [cited 2020 Oct 3]. Available from: https://www.who.int/healthpromotion/healthy-settings/en/

9. Promoting health in schools from evidence to action [Internet]. Available from: http://www.iuhpe.org/index.html?page=516&lang=en#sh_guidelines

10. Health-Promoting Schools. Regional guidelines development of health-promoting schools: A framework for action [Internet]. 1996 [cited 2020 Oct 10]. Available from: https://apps.who.int/iris/handle/10665/206847

11. Jain Y, Joshi N, Bhardwaj P, Suthar P. Health-promoting school in India: Approaches and challenges. *J Fam Med Prim Care.* 2019;8(10):3114.

12. Brown T, Moore TH, Hooper L, Gao Y, Zayegh A, Ijaz S, et al. Interventions for preventing obesity in children. Vol. 2019, *Cochrane Database of Systematic Reviews.* John Wiley and Sons Ltd; 2019.

13. Langford R, Bonell CP, Jones HE, Pouliou T, Murphy SM, Waters E, et al. The WHO health promoting school framework for improving the health and well-being of students and their academic achievement. Vol. 2014, *Cochrane Database of Systematic Reviews.* John Wiley and Sons Ltd; 2014.

14. Sutherland R, Nathan N, Brown A, Yoong S, Finch M, Lecathelinais C, et al. A randomized controlled trial to assess the potential efficacy, feasibility and acceptability of an m-health intervention targeting parents of school aged children to improve the nutritional quality of foods packed in the lunchbox "SWAP IT." *Int J Behav Nutr Phys Act.* 2019 Jul 2;16(1).

15. Shinde S, Weiss HA, Khandeparkar P, Pereira B, Sharma A, Gupta R, et al. A multicomponent secondary school health promotion intervention and adolescent health: An extension of the SEHER cluster randomised controlled trial in Bihar, India. *PLoS Med.* 2020 Feb 11;17(2):e1003021.

16. Perry CL, Stigler MH, Arora M, Reddy KS. Preventing tobacco use among young people in India: Project MYTRI. *Am J Public Health* 2010;99(5):899–906.

17. Brumana L, Arroyo A, Schwalbe NR, Lehtimaki S, Hipgrave DB. Maternal and child health services and an integrated, life-cycle approach to the prevention of noncommunicable diseases. *BMJ Glob Heal.* 2017;2(3): e000295.

18. Quintiliani L, Sattelmair J, Activity P, Sorensen G. The workplace as a setting for interventions to improve diet and promote physical activity. *World Heal Organ.* 2007;1–36.

19. Thakur J, Bains P, Kar S, Wadhwa S, Moirangthem P, Kumar R, et al. Integrated healthy workplace model: An experience from North Indian industry. *Indian J Occup Environ Med* [Internet]. 2012 Sep [cited 2020 Sep 30];16(3):108–13. Available from: /pmc/articles/PMC3683177/?report=abstract

20. Moy F, Sallam AAB, Wong M. The results of a worksite health promotion programme in Kuala Lumpur, Malaysia. *Health Promot Int.* 2006 Dec;21(4):301–10.

21. Chenworth D. Promoting employee well-being: Wellness strategies to improve health, performance and the bottom line. 2011;1–27. Available from: https://www.shrm.org/about/foundation/products/documents/6-11 promoting well being epg- final.pdf

22. Burton J. *Healthy Workplaces: A Model for Action.* 2010.

23. Chu AHY, Ng SHX, Tan CS, Win AM, Koh D, Müller-Riemenschneider F. A systematic review and meta-analysis of workplace intervention strategies to reduce sedentary time in white-collar workers. *Obes Rev* [Internet]. 2016 May 1 [cited 2020 Oct 4];17(5):467–81. Available from: http://doi.wiley.com/10.1111/obr.12388

24. Mulchandani R, Chandrasekaran AM, Shivashankar R, Kondal D, Agrawal A, Panniyammakal J, et al. Effect of workplace physical activity interventions on the cardio-metabolic health of working adults: Systematic review and meta-analysis. *Int J Behav Nutr Phys Act* 2019 Dec; 16(1): 1–6.

25. Morgan PJ, Collins CE, Plotnikoff RC, Cook AT, Berthon B, Mitchell S, et al. Efficacy of a workplace-based weight loss program for overweight male shift workers: The Workplace POWER (Preventing Obesity Without Eating like a Rabbit) randomized controlled trial. *Prev Med.* 2011 May 1;52(5):317–25.

26. Robroek SJW, van Lenthe FJ, van Empelen P, Burdorf A. Determinants of participation in worksite health promotion programmes: A systematic review. *Int J Behav Nutrit Phys Activity.* 2009; 6;26.

27. Atlantis E, Chow CM, Kirby A, Fiatarone Singh MA. Worksite intervention effects on physical health: A randomized controlled trial. *Health Promot Int.* 2006 Sep;21(3):191–200.

28. Vargas-Martínez AM, Romero-Saldaña M, De Diego-Cordero R. Economic evaluation of workplace health promotion interventions focused on Lifestyle: Systematic review and meta-analysis. *J Adv Nurs.* 2021;77(January):3657–91.

29. World Health Organization (WHO). Workplace health model [Internet]. [cited 2020 Oct 12]. Available from: https://www.cdc.gov/workplacehealthpromotion/model/index.html

30. World Health Organization (WHO). Healthy cities [Internet]. 2016 [cited 2020 Oct 3]. Available from: https://www.who.int/healthpromotion/healthy-cities/en/

31. Howard G, Bogh C, Prüss A, Goldstein G, Morgan J. Healthy Villages: A guide for communities and community health workers, *Appropriate Technology.* 2003 Jun 1; 30(2): 62.

32. World Health Organization (WHO). Shanghai consensus on healthy cities [Internet]. 2016. Available from: https://www.who.int/healthpromotion/conferences/9gchp/en/

33. Ministry of Health and Family Welfare (MOHFW). Improving the coverage and quality of village health and nutrition days [Internet]. New Delhi; 2012. Available from: https://www.intrahealth.org/sites/ihweb/files/files/media/improving-the-coverage-and-quality-of-village-health-and-nutrition-days/VHND_UP_30_10_12.pdf

34. Ministry of Health and Family Welfare (MOHFW). Handbook of the Village Health and Sanitation Committee [Internet]. Available from: https://nhm.gov.in/images/pdf/communitisation/vhsnc/Resources/Handbook_for_Members_of_VHSNC-English.pdf

35. Ministry of Health and Family Welfare (MOHFW). National health policy 2017: India [Internet]. 2012. Available from: https://www.nhp.gov.in//NHPfiles/national_health_policy_2017.pdf

36. AYUSHMAN BHARAT. Comprehensive primary health care through health and wellness centers [Internet]. New Delhi; 2018. Available from: http://nhsrcindia.org/sites/default/files/Operational Guidelines For Comprehensive Primary Health Care through Health and Wellness Centers.pdf

37. World Health Organization (WHO). Standards for health promotion in hospitals [Internet]. Available from: https://www.euro.who.int/__data/assets/pdf_file/0006/99762/e82490.pdf

38. WHO Europe. International network of health promoting hospitals and health services [Internet]. [cited 2020 Oct 29]. Available from: https://www.hphnet.org/about-us/

Case Study: *Public Health Suffers through Faulty Urban Constructions*

Malini Krishnankutty and Himanshu Burte

Modern urban planning emerged in the 19th-century European industrial city as a response to the public health crisis and led to better laid out streets and improvements in light and ventilation as well as water supply and sanitation. Since then, it is widely agreed that good urban policies and planning can actively help mitigate disease burdens and promote better health. Ironically, in the last two decades, it is urban policy and planning initiatives tied to urban renewal in Mumbai that have incubated public health disasters. Slum redevelopment projects and urban infrastructure projects undertaken in Mumbai since the early 2000s with resettlement policies, processes, and geographies are at the center of this public health crisis.

This crisis can be best illustrated through two specific instances, both located in the peripheral and poorly served M East and M West wards of Mumbai. The first is the discovery of a large number of tuberculosis cases in resettlement colonies for project-affected persons (PAPs) in Govandi West, located near Mumbai's oldest landfill site in 2017. The second is the widespread morbidity in the Slum Redevelopment Authority (SRA) township at Mahul, a site close to a heavily industrialized zone, leading to a long protest by its residents since 2018. Each of these sites is home to around 30,000 people. The spatiality of the resettlement colonies is at the center of the public health crises in both cases: the dangerous location in proximity to highly polluted areas (heavy industries and landfill sites), and the specific design of the residential layout causing overcrowding and inadequate light and ventilation. Densities here are more than twice the National Building Code–suggested maximum of 500 tenements/hectare. Tenement size is uniformly 269 square feet and the average family size is 5.

Mahul was deliberately zoned and reserved for hazardous industries in the first Development Plan 1964 (DP 1964) for Mumbai. It houses heavy industries, such as fertilizer factories, oil refineries, and a thermal power plant, and abuts an atomic energy research facility. DP 1964 had specified a very low Floor Space Index (FSI; the ratio of total permissible built-up area on a plot to the total plot area of 0.5 for the entire ward). This was half of the permitted FSI in other suburbs to intentionally keep the residential density low. Planners believe that FSI helps control the population in a given area and thus a low FSI would help minimize the number of people exposed to risks of possible industrial disasters and pollution exposure. The first dilution of this precautionary approach has been the steady increase of FSI in the M ward over the years in response to the pressure for real estate development in the city.

Since 1995, new slum housing policies have been introduced by the state that incentivizes the market provision of free housing for slum dwellers through various 'relaxations' of the existing development control regulations. Housing for PAPs was also incentivized under these policies. Under one such PAP scheme, the Mahul township, consisting of over 70 seven-story buildings and more than 17,000 flats, was built between 2011 and 2017 by a private developer to house PAPs.[1] It was originally conceived to receive people displaced by the Brihanmumbai stormwater drainage project. Since then, however, PAPs affected by various other infrastructure projects in the city have been moved there.[2] The refineries and the atomic energy facility had opposed the location of the project, citing security concerns due to the location being so close to sensitive installations. In response, the Supreme Court directed in 2013 that some buildings situated nearest to the existing industrial facilities be handed over to the Mumbai police. As a result, a few buildings are for Mumbai police housing, though police families subsequently have refused to move into these flats.[3]

Resettled families in Mahul have faced tremendous illness burdens in the form of respiratory and skin diseases. A 2013 survey by the Environment Pollution Research Center (EPRC) of King Edward Memorial Hospital recorded that '67% of the residents in Mahul complained of breathlessness more than three times a month, 86.6% suffered from eye irritation and 84.5% reported a choking sensation due to bad air quality.'[4] This report, along with the Maharashtra Pollution Control Board's 2014 air sample analyses indicating high levels of toluene, formed the basis of the National Green Tribunal's judgment of 2015 which held that Mahul was 'unfit for human habitation,' since all the symptoms displayed by the residents matched those caused by exposure to toluene diisocyanate, a possible carcinogen that is toxic even in low concentrations. The decision to resettle large numbers of people so close to polluting areas in Mahul flouts the most basic principle of planning of avoiding harm to human health, especially by avoiding locating 'conflicting' uses such as a polluting industry and housing near each other. Planning and policy decisions like this

 DOI: 10.1201/b23385-24

can both trigger crises that undo past efforts with resettled communities and present steep challenges to future ones related to mitigating public health burdens. This underlines how intertwined human health is with a healthy environment and good policy: if either of them is compromised, it can negatively impact human health.

In addition to the issue of hazardous location, the residents' health is further compromised due to aspects of the site layout and building design at both the Mahul and Govandi resettlement housing schemes, both traceable to the steep increase in population density – well beyond the maximum specified by the National Building Code (NBC) – enabled by a sanctioned exception to the Development Control Regulations (DCRs) applicable in the city. The exception was first introduced by the state government into the DCRs of the Mumbai DP 1991 to enable the redevelopment of slums through private participation, by accommodating existing slum dwellers in buildings on the same site and building additional apartments for sale to cross-subsidize the former. This regulatory exception (or 'relaxation') thus instituted overcrowding for economic reasons – to enable profits for private developers undertaking redevelopment. The SRA, a parastatal organization, was created to regulate all slum redevelopment projects. Interestingly, the resettlement colony design was also brought under the regulation of the SRA with the relaxations in regulations mentioned earlier. Among these relaxations was an increase in the number of tenements that could be built per hectare. Initially, 500 dwelling units (du)/hectare was the *maximum* permissible in the NBC. However, the relaxation modified this by making 500 du/hectare the *minimum* permissible under existing DCRs, with an accompanying reduction in the minimum open space to be left between buildings (to enable natural light and ventilation in every apartment) that still apply to all other housing projects in the rest of the city. These relaxations allowed more people to be packed into available land for resettlement colonies. The resulting situation would qualify as 'overcrowding' under the NBC, which is a non-statutory code but has long been the template for all building codes in Indian cities so as to guarantee a minimally healthful and habitable built environment. Naturally, this has possibly led to serious health consequences.

At Govandi's resettlement colonies at Lallubhai Compound and Natwar Parekh, a recent study[5] shockingly found that the prevalence of tuberculosis (TB) in the planned PAP resettlement colonies was the same as in the 'unplanned' slums of M (E) ward.[6] In fact, a majority of the patients reported that they contacted the disease after they moved into the resettlement colonies. The study established a strong correlation between the incidence of TB and the excessive density and constrained design of individual buildings and the arrangement of buildings on site. An important driver is possibly the inadequate open space left between adjacent building blocks, which makes adequate daylight and natural ventilation impossible in the overcrowded individual apartments (25 sq m each, average family size 5.27 per unit). In both Govandi layouts, seven-storied housing blocks run parallel to each other with only a 3 m open space between them. The study found that TB cases clustered around particular locations in the colony marked by extremely poor indoor daylight and the number of air changes per hour in the tenements. These typically were on the lower floors of the buildings and in the long apartment blocks that were in the middle of an array of linear buildings.[7]

Importantly, though they are effectively urban planning interventions, neither resettlement program has been worked out through the statutory land-use planning process, though provisions for PAPs have been part of DPs 1964 and 1991.[8] The key measures that have resulted in the public health crisis can be considered examples of 'sovereign planning',[9] that is, planning action that is not initiated or directed by trained planners within the state but enacted by the bureaucratic-political decision-making establishment that controls urban planning at the state-government level. Clearly, whoever makes planning decisions needs to be trained rigorously in their public health implications to avoid the kind of outcomes discussed herein.

NOTES

1. Sayed N and Mapakwar C, 'Police to get 2000 flats in Chembur buildings they opposed,' *Mumbai Mirror*, 1 September 13, https://mumbaimirror.indiatimes.com/mumbai/crime/police-to-get-2000-flats-in-chembur-bldgs-they-opposed/articleshow/22193147.cms

2. The Mumbai Metropolitan Region Development Authority (MMRDA) obtained 30 buildings with some 4000 tenements in Mahul for resettlement of PAPs from various transport and road infrastructure projects in Powai, Ghatkopar, Chembur, Vakola, and Bandra (E). The Municipal Corporation of Greater Mumbai (MCGM) relocated about 5000 families displaced when settlements along the Tansa pipeline were cleared, following a high court order.

3. One of the buildings is now slated to be used as a godown for confiscated goods by the police. Naik Y, 'Flats for cops to be converted into godown, Mumbai police finally admits it has failed to convince cops to move to Mahul,' *Mumbai Mirror*, 9 May 2019, https://mumbai-mirror.indiatimes.com/mumbai/other/flats-for-policemen-to-be-converted-into-godown/articleshow/69243248.cms

4. Kappal B, 'Life and death in Mumbai's "human dumping ground,"' *LiveMint*, 28 September 2018, https://www.livemint.com/Leisure/Ki7VXzsgdtebWpHmXQPuMI/Life-and-death-in-Mumbais-human-dumping-ground.html

5. Pardeshi P, Balaram Jadhav B, Singh R, Kapoor N, Bardhan R, Jana A, David S, and Roy N, 'Association between architectural parameters and burden of tuberculosis in three resettlement colonies of M-East Ward, Mumbai, India, *Cities & Health*, 2020.

6. Incidentally, M (E) has the highest TB incidence among all the 24 wards in Mumbai.

7. Interestingly, through a comparison with a comparable resettlement colony, the study did find a role for architectural design that mitigated the deleterious effects of planning 'relaxations' that increased density and minimized distance between buildings.

8. The DPs – the only statutory instrument of urban planning in Indian cities – are devised by urban local bodies, which are democratically elected and, in theory, politically accountable to citizens. However, two of the most important initiatives of urban renewal – slum redevelopment, and infrastructure building and upgradation – that displaced people were directed by parastatals such as the SRA and MMRDA, which are not politically accountable to the local population and report directly to the state government.

9. Krishnankutty, M, 'Fragmentary planning and spaces of opportunity in peri-urban Mumbai,' *Economic and Political Weekly*, 53(12): 68–75, 24 March 2018.

14 Public Health Approaches to Healthy Behaviors among Children and Adolescents in Schools

Tina Rawal, Surbhi Shrivastava, Chetna Duggal, and Melissa Blythe Harrell

CONTENTS

> No education system can be effective unless it promotes the health and well-being of its students, staff and community.
>
> **Tedros Ghebreyesus, director-general, World Health Organization; and Audrey Azoulay, director-general, UNESCO**

INTRODUCTION

Child and adolescent health play a vital role in the development of a country. Although adolescence and young adulthood are generally considered healthy times of life, several important health problems either start or peak during these years. Behaviors and conditions related to risk factors often coexist in the same individual adding a cumulative risk for their poor health. Many of these are precursors and determinants of noncommunicable diseases (NCDs), mental health and neurological disorders, and injuries, which place a heavy burden, in terms of adult mortality, morbidity, disability, and socioeconomic losses, on the world in general, and low- and middle-income (LMICs) countries in particular.

The current health status of children and adolescents in LMICs has improved but is still dismal with major inequalities existing within and across countries. As such, Article 24 and related articles of the United Nations Convention on the Rights of the Child (1990) recognize that every child has a right to the "highest attainable standard of health". To this end, the World Health Organization (WHO) adopted the coordinated school health program (CSHP) under its health promoting schools (HPSs) initiative to represent key settings through which health can be improved (1) (Figure 14.1).

Since then, the CSHP has evolved in tandem with our understanding of the socioecological (2) paradigms of health (Figure 14.2), which explore the interrelationship between social systems or settings and human health. In 2008, Lohrmann provided a comprehensive version of the CHSP based on public health and child development theories that incorporate the influence of personal

DOI: 10.1201/b23385-25

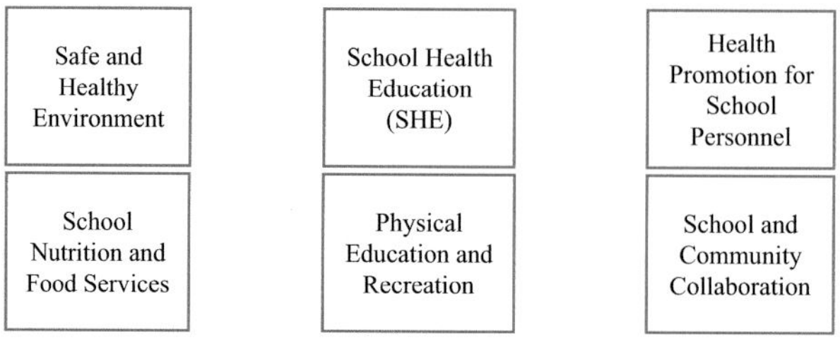
Safe and Healthy Environment
School Health Education (SHE)
Health Promotion for School Personnel
School Nutrition and Food Services
Physical Education and Recreation
School and Community Collaboration

Figure 14.1 Six essential components of health promoting schools.

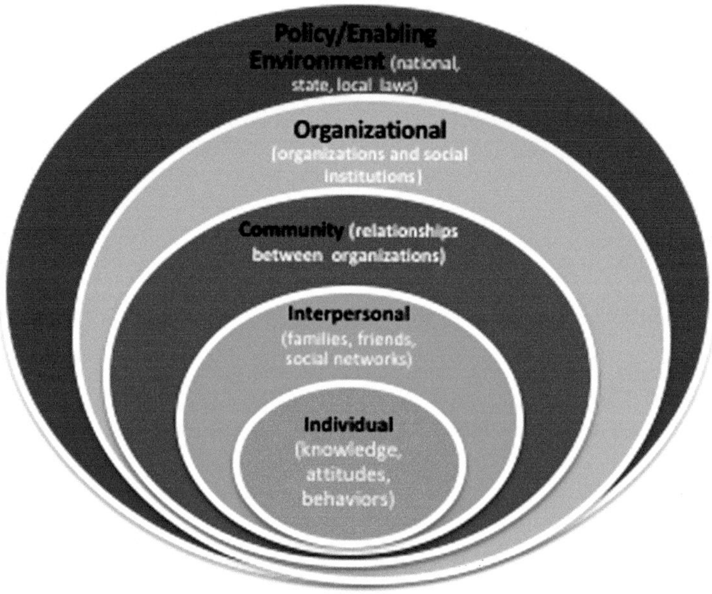

Figure 14.2 The social-ecological model: a framework for prevention.

and social environments on health behavior, along with models that incorporate the influence of ecology (3). Altogether, these provide a robust framework within which discussions about school health programs in this chapter will be grounded.

WHO and UNESCO consequently launched a new initiative – "Making Every School a Health Promoting School" – by developing and promoting global standards for HPS. One of the priorities identified was to establish systems for collecting better data, monitoring, reporting, providing evidence, and utilizing that evidence to make policy and plan implementation.

OVERVIEW OF STRATEGIES FOR HEALTH PROMOTING SCHOOLS

Health promotion in a school setting includes comprehensive programs/approaches/strategies that can effectively encourage children to adopt healthy behaviors and/or refrain from unhealthy ones. The strategies may focus on individuals, groups, and communities to bring behavior change and support in:

- Creating a supportive environment by building healthy policies (e.g., canteen policy)
- Adopting multicomponent and collective action to empower and build skills

This chapter captures specific components of child and adolescent health, as covered by most adolescent health-related programs, like RKSK (Rashtriya Kishor Swasthya Karyakram), in India, namely, nutrition and physical activity, tobacco and alcohol use, environmental risks, mental health, and oral health. Each component is introduced with a *problem statement* that highlights the prevalence of relevant risk factors and disease conditions in LMICs. Thereafter, public health approaches with best practices from LMIC countries are presented *in focus*. This chapter concludes with a set of *key takeaways* that can inform policy and programmatic interventions in the school setting.

NUTRITION AND PHYSICAL ACTIVITY

Nutrition plays an important role to support the proper growth of children and adolescents. At the same time, malnutrition may adversely affect their growth and development including impaired cognitive behavior, NCDs, and communicable diseases among children and adolescents.

Problem Statement

Malnutrition is a major public health challenge in LMICs. India currently faces a paradoxical co-occurrence of under- and overweight/obesity. Environmental factors and lifestyle choices, including urbanization, play major roles in the rising prevalence of malnutrition among children and adolescents. Overweight and obese children are more likely to grow into obese adults, who in turn are at higher risk for developing NCDs. The school environment has the potential to inculcate healthy living habits from an early age and balance these by varying rural and urban contexts and income inequalities.

In Focus: India

The ongoing efforts of India's Ministry of Health and Family Welfare (MoHFW) to improve nutrition among children and adolescents include the Mid-Day Meal Scheme, the school health program under Ayushman Bharat, and the Food Safety and Standards Authority of India's Safe and Nutritious Food at School program.

> The Mid-Day Meal Scheme (MDMS) was launched by the Government of India (GoI) in August 1995 as a National Programme of Nutritional Support to Primary Education (NP-NSPE) (14). The program aims to provide at least one-third of recommended calories and half of the proteins to every beneficiary daily. Primary school children (classes I–V) attending government and government-aided schools are provided a free supply of 100 grams of food grains per school day. The Honorable Supreme Court of India ordered the GoI in 2001 that the NP-NSPE should provide 'cooked meals' with a minimum nutritive content of 300 calories and 8–12 grams of protein for each day of school for a minimum of 200 days. The scheme was extended to cover children of upper primary classes (i.e., classes VI–VIII) in 2007 by the GoI and changed its name to National Programme of Mid-Day Meal in Schools (NP-MDMS) with a revised nutritional norm of 700 calories and 20 grams of protein. Since 2008, the NP-MDMS has been implemented across the country. NP-MDMS has been reported as one of the successful entitlement schemes of the GoI and has resulted in an increase in enrollment, attendance, and retention of children in schools and helped foster social equality and enhanced gender equity.

Additionally, "Diabetes Awareness and Prevention Education", a school-based intervention, was implemented in Delhi over a period of two years to enhance knowledge and positively alter attitudes toward healthy lifestyle practices (4). The program strategies included the following: training teachers to facilitate innovative classroom activities; training students to become peer leaders; five interactive classroom curricula; teacher-led discussions; peer-led small-group activities; and creative and age-appropriate components of the educational modules such as fun learning games, students' worksheets, and intraschool competitions (e.g., poster-making) as an extension of the classroom activities. Evaluation of this intervention demonstrated a significant increase in the knowledge about diabetes and its risk factors among school students, and daily consumption of vegetables and fruits significantly increased among government (public) school students to 76.4% after intervention from 68.3% at baseline ($p = 0.003$). Students from both government and private schools showed a reduction in the consumption of carbonated drinks, fried snacks, sweets, and chips after intervention among both boys and girls, and more children reported going out and playing with friends during their leisure time (44.1% after intervention vs. 35.1% students at baseline)

ENVIRONMENTAL RISKS

A safe physical environment is a prerequisite for effective learning, the absence of which can have direct effects on the health of school-going adolescents. Some key environmental risks include air pollution, lack of water and inadequate sanitation, and road traffic injuries (RTIs). Moreover, LMICs account for 93% of child road traffic deaths.

Problem Statement

The exposure of children to $PM_{2.5}$ through solid fuels in India is 285 μg/m^3, which is greatly more than the WHO guideline of 35 μg/m^3 or the Indian standard of 40 μg/m^3 (5). Moreover, water, sanitation, and hygiene (WASH) facilities in schools are poorly maintained, allowing an unhygienic and unsafe school environment (6). Among those aged 10–14 years in India, RTIs are the leading cause of death (7). Furthermore, the highest burden of injuries and fatalities in developing countries is borne disproportionately by poor people, as they are mostly pedestrians, cyclists, and passengers of buses and minibuses.

In Focus: Egypt

Between 2007 and 2014, about 200,000 schoolchildren in over 370 primary schools were reached through the hygiene awareness campaign in the governorates of Assiut, Sohag, and Qena in Egypt (8). This effort included capacity-building for 2000 staff members who conducted future awareness activities. Child-to-child, child-to-parents, and parents-to-community approaches were adopted as entry points for better sanitation and hygiene practices. Findings showed that factors for the successful implementation of a school health program that addresses environmental risks and hygiene and sanitation include: multisectoral convergence (such as Ministries of Health, Education, Agriculture, Finance); multistakeholder support (e.g., involvement of community members, parents, and guardians); and participation of children.

In Focus: Republic of Korea

To address the problem of pedestrians suffering death and injury at the expense of wider, faster roads, the Korean government carried out an analysis of RTI records and the highest-risk locations in the network (9). A new national strategy was adopted to improve road safety through investments in school zone programs, improving the regulation of school buses, increasing fines for violations within school zones, clamping down on unregulated school transport, supporting civil society organizations in road safety advocacy, and continuously amending and improving road safety legislation. These multilevel interventions have reportedly contributed to a 95% reduction in RTIs among children under 14 years of age between 1998 and 2012.

TOBACCO AND ALCOHOL USE

Tobacco is the single largest preventable cause of death the world over and a growing public health concern for present and future generations. The most susceptible time for initiating and experimenting with tobacco use is during adolescence and young adulthood.

Problem Statement

According to the Global Adult Tobacco Survey (GATS) India, 2017, the prevalence of current tobacco use in any form among adults is 28.6%. As per the Global Youth Tobacco Survey (GYTS), the current use in any form among students aged 13–15 years is 8.5%. Globally, school surveys indicated alcohol use starts before the age of 15 years, and the per capita consumption of alcohol in those over 15 years old has increased from 5.5 liters in 2005 to 6.4 liters in 2016. In India, the prevalence of current alcohol use in children (10–17 years) is 1.3% (10).

In Focus: India

Project MYTRI (Mobilizing Youth for Tobacco Related Initiatives in India; 2001–2006), a school-based group randomized trial among sixth- to ninth-grade students in 32 schools in two Indian cities (n = 16 in Delhi and n = 16 in Chennai), was conducted with a long-term goal to prevent and reduce tobacco use among young people. The program involved four primary components: (i) 13 sessions of classroom curricula across 2 years; (ii) school posters; (iii) parental involvement (postcards were sent home to parents); and (iv) peer-led health activism (peer leadership component). MYTRI demonstrated the effectiveness of school-based interventions in reducing tobacco use among Indian students by reducing current tobacco use, reducing their future intentions to use tobacco, and by enhancing their health advocacy skills. Overall, current tobacco use increased by 68% in the control group and decreased by 17% in the intervention group over the study duration. Intentions to smoke increased by 5% in the control group, whereas intentions to smoke decreased in intervention schools by 11%. Intentions to chew tobacco decreased by 12% in the control group but decreased by 28% in the intervention group. Changes in students' (a) knowledge about the negative health effects of tobacco, (b) beliefs about its social consequences, (c) reasons to use tobacco, (d) reasons not to use tobacco, (e) advocacy skills/self-efficacy, and (f) normative beliefs about tobacco use were significantly associated with reductions in students' intentions to use tobacco and tobacco use behaviors.

The study provided robust research evidence and was adopted by the MoHFW for up-scaling at the national level. As a result, school health programs form a key component of the National Tobacco Control Programme (NTCP) that was launched in 2007. The GoI scaled up school health interventions incorporating tobacco use prevention lessons or curricula like Project MYTRI in all schools across the country (11).

MENTAL HEALTH

Children and adolescents can present with a range of neuropsychiatric disorders and psychosocial concerns (e.g., depression, anxiety). Apart from genetic vulnerability, adverse environmental factors, such as conflict within the family and bullying in school, can put children and adolescents at a higher risk of developing mental health concerns.

Problem Statement

The prevalence rate of child and adolescent psychiatric disorders such as neurodevelopmental disorders, depression, anxiety-related disorders, and so on in India has been reported to be 6%–7% in the community and around 20% in schools (12). The National Mental Health Survey (2016) by the National Institute for Mental Health and Neurosciences (NIMHANS) found the prevalence of psychological disorders among adolescents at 7.3% (13). Neuropsychiatric conditions are the leading cause of disability among young people. Poor mental health outcomes in children and adolescents further impact their developmental and educational outcomes and are also linked to substance abuse, violence, etc., severely impacting their potential for living happy and productive lives. Moreover, in India, suicide is the leading cause of death in the age group of 15–29 years. India's contribution to global suicide deaths has been reported as 36.6% for women and 24.3% for men (14). Therefore, suicide is a serious mental health concern in India and also requires urgent public health attention.

In Focus: India

The GoI initiated the National Mental Health Programme. In 2011, the Policy Group appointed by the MoHFW recommended including child mental health services at district hospitals and recommended preventive and promotive services such as a suicide prevention program and life skills education in schools for children and adolescents. The Rashtriya Bal Swasthya Karyakram (RBSK) was launched by the MoHFW in 2014 and includes a focus on early identification and early intervention for development delays including disability in children from birth to 18 years. There is a huge treatment gap in Indian mental health care due to a range of political, social, cultural, and economic factors, and there is an urgent need to develop and implement contextually relevant community-based models that include schools as a health promoting setting.

In Focus: Singapore

To support school-going students with mental health problems, the Response, Early Intervention and Assessment in Community Mental Health (REACH) program was developed in Singapore (15). This community-based model helps build the capacities of schools and community partners to detect and manage mental health problems to provide quality care that is effective, accessible, timely, affordable, and safe for children and their families. The evaluation of the program revealed that this community-based model was more cost-effective as compared to hospital-based care, and children showed a significant reduction in psychosocial concerns and improvement in prosocial behaviors after six months.

ORAL HEALTH

The years of adolescence (10–19 years) offer an ideal window for building the foundations of adolescent health, including but not limited to oral health. Risk factors for oral diseases include unhealthy diet, tobacco use, alcohol use, and poor oral hygiene.

Problem Statement

Oral diseases such as dental caries (tooth decay), periodontal diseases (gum diseases), and tooth loss have emerged as major public health problems in the South-East Asia Region. Especially for children and adolescents, those suffering from poor oral health are 12 times more likely to have more restricted-activity days, including missing school, than those who do not.

In Focus: Thailand

Evidence supports strengthening the integration of oral health into universal health coverage (UHC) (16). Thailand has successfully implemented UHC and provided evidence of such integration. Although the models of oral health promotion with extensive school-based supervised brushing and fissure sealant programs have been well accepted in Thailand, a gap has been identified in the participation of "significant others", such as school teachers (17). The research project has demonstrated that the use of fluoridated toothpaste administered by schoolteachers and undertaken within the context of an enhanced school oral health program has positive effects in terms of reduction in caries.

KEY TAKEAWAYS: PROGRAM AND POLICY INTERVENTIONS

- There is a need for a holistic health policy action to integrate school health programs into health promotion and prevention of lifestyle-related diseases in effective ways to foster a healthy environment.
- A multicomponent approach working at various levels of the socioecological model is paramount for holistically addressing environmental risks.
- Importance should be placed on behavior change cost-effective interventions in school environments with the availability of supportive infrastructure that can facilitate the uptake of healthier practices at various levels. This includes the availability of adequate facilities, physical and psychosocial support, screenings, referrals, and provision of school-based health and nutrition services, which have impacts on improved education outcomes.
- Building capacities and communications of school staff along with other stakeholders including parents would strengthen networks to support young people's health.
- Community-based, child-friendly, and youth-oriented approaches need to be implemented to provide quality care that is accessible and affordable through culturally relevant and participatory activities.

LIST OF ACRONYMS

CSHP: Coordinated school health program
GATS: Global Adult Tobacco Survey
GoI: Government of India
HIV/AIDS: Human immunodeficiency virus/acquired immune deficiency syndrome
HPSs: Health promoting schools
LMICs: Low- and middle-income countries
MoHFW: Ministry of Health and Family Welfare
MYTRI: Mobilizing Youth for Tobacco Related Initiatives
NCDs: Noncommunicable diseases
NIMHANS: National Institute for Mental Health and Neurosciences
NTCP: National Tobacco Control Programme
$PM_{2.5}$: Particulate $matter_{2.5}$
RBSK: Rashtriya Bal Swasthya Karyakram
REACH: Response, Early Intervention and Assessment in Community Mental Health
RKSK: Rashtriya Kishor Swasthya Karyakram
RTIs: Road traffic injuries
UHC: Universal health coverage
WASH: Water, sanitation, and hygiene
WHO: World Health Organization

REFERENCES

1. WHO SEARO. A guide for establishing health promoting schools in the South-East Asia Region. 2003. Available from: https://apps.who.int/iris/handle/10665/204729.

2. Townsend N, Foster C. Developing and applying a socio-ecological model to the promotion of healthy eating in the school. *Public Health Nutr.* 2013;16(6):1101–8.

3. Lohrmann DK. A complementary ecological model of the coordinated school health program. *Public Health Rep.* 2008;123(6):695–703.

4. Bassi S, Gupta VK, Chopra I, Ranjani H, Saligram N, Arora M. Novel school-based health intervention program: A step toward early diabetes prevention. *Int J Diabetes Dev Countries.* 2015;35(4):460–8.

5. Welfare MoHaF. *Report of the Steering Committee on Air Pollution and Health Related Issues.* 2015 Available from: http://theasthmafiles.ss.uci.edu/sites/default/files/artifacts/media/pdf/report_of_the_steering_committee_on_air_pollution_and_health_related_issues_ministry_of_health_family_welfare.pdf.

6. Fansa W. Leave no one behind: Voices of women, adolescent girls, elderly, persons with disabilities and sanitation workforce. *India Country Report.* 2015. Available from: https://www.wsscc.org/sites/default/files/uploads/2016/08/Leave-No-One-Behind-Nepal-Country-report.pdf.

7. The George Institute for Global Health India. Preventing road traffic injuries in school-going children. 2015. Available from: https://www.georgeinstitute.org.in/philanthropic-opportunities/preventing-road-traffic-injuries-in-school-going-children.

8. UNICEF Egypt. Water, sanitation and hygiene. 2017. Available from: https://www.unicef.org/egypt/water-sanitation-and-hygiene#_ftn1.

9. World Health Organization. *Global Status Report on Road Safety.* 2018. Available from: https://www.who.int/publications/i/item/9789241565684.

10. India Ministry of Social Justice and Empowerment. Magnitude of substance use in India. 2019. Available from: http://ndusindia.in/downloads/Magnitude_India_EXEUCTIVE_SUMMARY.pdf.

11. Arora M, Stigler MH, Srinath Reddy K. Effectiveness of health promotion in preventing tobacco use among adolescents in India: Research evidence informs the National Tobacco Control Programme in India. *Global Health Promotion.* 2011;18(1):09–12.

12. World Health Organization. Risks to mental health: An overview of vulnerabilities and risk factors. 2012. Available from: https://cdn.who.int/media/docs/default-source/mental-health/risks_to_mental_health_en_27_08_12.pdf?sfvrsn=44f5907d_10&download=true.

13. Gururaj G, Varghese M, Benegal V, Rao G, Pathak K, Singh L, et al. National Mental Health Survey of India: Summary. Bengaluru: National Institute of Mental Health and Neurosciences. 2016:1–48.

14. Dandona R, Kumar GA, Dhaliwal RS, Naghavi M, Vos T, Shukla DK, Vijayakumar L, Gururaj G, Thakur JS, Ambekar A, Sagar R. Gender differentials and state variations in suicide deaths in India: The global burden of disease study 1990–2016. *Lancet Public Health.* 2018;3(10):e478–e89.

15. Lim CG, Loh H, Renjan V, Tan J, Fung D. Child community mental health services in Asia Pacific and Singapore's REACH model. *Brain Sci.* 2017;7(10):126.

16. Mathur MR, Williams DM, Reddy KS, Watt RG. Universal health coverage: A unique policy opportunity for oral health. *J Dent Res.* 2015;94(3 Suppl) Suppl:3S–5S.

17. Petersen PE, Hunsrisakhun J, Thearmontree A, Pithpornchaiyakul S, Hintao J, Jürgensen N, et al. School-based intervention for improving the oral health of children in southern Thailand. *Community Dent Health.* 2015;32(1):44–50.

Case Study: *"UDAAN: Towards a Better Future ...," an Adolescent Education Program in Jharkhand*

Aprajita Gogoi

School-based adolescent education programs, especially those that combine comprehensive reproductive health education and life-skills-based education, hold great promise in promoting health knowledge, attitudes, and behaviors for in-school adolescents. The Government of Jharkhand initiated an adolescent education program in the year 2006. The program in the state was named 'UDAAN: Towards a Better...' Since 2007, the Jharkhand Council for Education Research and Training, under the Department of School Education and Literacy, has been designated as the lead implementing agency for the program in the state. The Centre for Catalyzing Change has been providing technical support with help from the David and Lucile Packard Foundation. Udaan exemplifies collaboration across the sectors and this multistakeholder model underscores government–NGO partnership to empower adolescents through the school system.

The state education department leads the program with technical support from the Centre for Catalyzing Change. Major strategies include the State Core Committee providing policy and strategic directions; a state-level nodal officer from State Education Services has been designated to extend necessary coordination and administrative support. Other health promotion strategies include teacher-delivered, state-specific, and age-appropriate sexual and reproductive health and rights (SRHR) curricula; systematic and quality training of nodal teachers; multistakeholder involvement; sustained advocacy for community buy-in and acceptance; promoting life skills activities through student-led Udaan clubs; mainstreaming of content in pre-service and in-services teachers' training system and integration of adolescent education content in school textbooks for sustainability; monitoring and supervision by key functionaries from education department; fiscal contribution by education and health departments; and the Packard Foundation's long-term support to the Centre for Catalyzing Change for providing technical support.

Students attending the program are aware of sexual and reproductive health and have started accessing National Adolescent Health Program services at 'adolescent friendly health clinics' known as 'YUVA Maitri Kendra' in the state. In August 2010, the program was introduced to all 203 residential Kasturba Gandhi Balika Vidyalayas (KGBVs). Later, in the year 2014, an innovative digital adolescent education package was introduced in these residential KGBVs and 68 private schools in the state to supplement the implementation of Udaan.

Findings of periodical assessments show that the program met the gaps through the aforesaid strategies, leading to improved knowledge, attitudes, and life skills in critical areas such as SRHR, gender equality, changes during adolescence, and HIV/AIDS. Overall, trends show 57.5% of students reporting positive self-efficacy and 49.5% students with high leadership skills; a 16% increase over baseline was observed among students identifying puberty changes; 72% of teachers were comfortable conducting sessions on adolescence; and 49.6% of students were aware of more than three modes of HIV transmission and 45.4% were aware of more than three ways of prevention besides correct age at marriage for girls and boys. Udaan alumni also demonstrated correct knowledge of sexual harassment by identifying correct descriptions of sexual harassment, the legal age of marriage for boys as 21 and 18 for girls, and ways to handle negative peer pressure and show gender-equitable views.

Udaan is an example of how an intersectoral health program is institutionalized and led successfully by the Department of Education. An age-appropriate and state-specific sexual and reproductive health curricula, sustained advocacy, quality training, and convergence between line departments have made it a sustainable program that reaches 1,100,000 students during the program life course. Udaan was selected as a "Good and Replicable Practices and Innovations in Public Healthcare System" in 2016 by the Ministry of Health and Family Welfare (MoHFW), Government of India. Also in 2016, the World Health Organization chose to document this model as a first-generation at-scale adolescent education program from the South East Asia region with an intent to disseminate it globally. MoHFW, in its 'Revised National RKSK Guidelines 2018,' acknowledged Udaan as a successful model of convergence.

 DOI: 10.1201/b23385-26

Case Study: *Using Creative Arts for Health Promotion*

Mallika Sarabhai and Suneet Singh Puri

Using the performing arts to reflect upon social issues has been at the helm of Darpana's monumental body of work. From as early as the 1960s, Mrinalini Sarabhai – the founder of Darpana – began to push the boundaries of tradition and use the myriad language of Indian classical dance to tell stories of the social evils that plagued Indian society. Through her dance, she became one of the foremost proponents – of the newly independent India – to use the performing arts to charter a more progressive, inclusive, and healthy path toward nation-building.

Over the years, Darpana began to evolve: expanding its repertoire to include Gujarati theatre and puppetry, while the Darpana Performing Group continued to tour India and the world with an array of compelling stories – contemporary to their time – with a strong focus on women, highlighting social evils and rituals, maternal and prenatal health, women empowerment, and sexual and reproductive health and rights to name a few. An example of this was when Darpana's puppeteers started working with the Central Ministry of Rural Development in teaching village women the benefits of using a smokeless stove. From the 1980s onward, Darpana began a phase of transformation – inspired by Vikram Sarabhai's vision and belief – wherein technological intervention could facilitate effective communication. The power to use the medium as the message[1] in spreading knowledge and informing people about healthy habits, perils of superstition, and gendered misunderstandings was understood and promulgated by both Vikram and Mrinalini Sarabhai. With their legacy and knowledge, Darpana stepped forth to marry the innovations of technology with the emotional intelligence of the arts in creating an innovative formula to reach people and affect change. Darpana focused on creating behavior change communication (BCC) through the arts and collaborating with the government and nongovernmental organizations (NGOs) to educate the public on issues of health, education, and empowering women.

Darpana has used the arts to mediate health communication for several decades. One of the earliest experiences was in creating a series of one-minute films on hygiene, malaria, and the necessity for vaccination for the Ahmedabad Municipal Corporation in 1980. Since then, issues addressed include infant and maternal health, HIV/AIDS, malaria, diabetes, cervical cancer, and the need for hand washing with soap after defecation.[2]

Darpana strongly believes in the ability of the performing arts to act as a bridge to reduce differences between people from different backgrounds and communicate at a more human level – through emotions.

Darpana designed and began operating using different levels of methodological intervention, creating a structural framework to categorize the different approaches of BCC.

1. Peer-educator and training: The arts have immense capacity in building a sense of equality in society, encouraging people to find their voice, reinforcing people's sense of pride in their community, and making people more responsible for their society.[3] In order to achieve this, we had to work closely with individuals from target communities and train them to be actor-activists to communicate effectively using storytelling mediums anchored in uniquely designed performing arts techniques. Darpana has conducted projects across districts in Gujarat, with UNICEF, Population Services International (PSI), and the Gujarat AIDS Society, to name a few, training more than 200 peer-educators on a variety of subjects such as HIV/AIDS that had a deep-seated impact in the target communities.

2. Training local folk artists: Darpana selects folk performers from the target community and helps them adapt their art by keeping intact their vernacular language, culture, and style. Darpana also helps the performers create new performances, sending them back to the community as activists with particular messages or learning. The trained local artists then perform in their communities and co-opt other community influencers as peer-educators, who eventually become harbingers of change at the family and societal levels. Having a wide range of experience across different states – Gujarat, Jharkhand, Maharashtra, Rajasthan, Assam, and Chhattisgarh, to name a few – and working with different sets of artists and art forms (Bhavai,[4] Bharud,[5] and other folk art forms), Darpana has been able to keep the fundamental principle of connecting with people through emotion intact. Themes addressed range from HIV/AIDS awareness, to educating communities against witch-hunting, maternal and infant health, diabetes, cervical cancer check-ups and treatment, and basic hygiene practices.

DOI: 10.1201/b23385-27

3. Darpana's most significant expertise lies in creating powerful, compelling performances thoroughly researched by engaging with real-world scenarios affecting citizens. The performances cater to a privileged class of audience: private corporations, government officers, senior counsel and judges, diplomats (foreign and national), and other such influential people. Many of the hugely successful shows such as *Sita's Daughters* (performed 600 shows across the world) highlighted issues around women's health and female feticide in India.

Behavior change is much harder than the simplistic notion of preventive messaging. Changing mindsets requires a connection with people at an interpersonal level. Print media can be effective if people know how to read, but in situations and places where illiteracy is high and the reach of broadcast is low, interpersonal means of communication such as using performing arts can be very effective.

Darpana believes that posing alternative realities through arts interventions allows audiences to be educated to make their own informed decisions. This gives them an onus to affect change in mindsets, allowing for the possibility of permanent behavior change.

NOTES

1. Marshall McLuhan, "Medium Is the Message," accessed March 25, 2019, https://www.youtube.com/watch?v=UoCrx0scCkM.

2. "Killi Anandachi," n.d.

3. "UNICEF Peer Educator Project," n.d., Children in Gujarat | UNICEF India

4. "Bhavai is a popular folk theatre form in Gujarat with a 700-year old history. ... Bhavai's original aim was mass awareness and entertainment; hence it evolved to have an open-air style, with simple storylines and exaggerated acting." Prateeksha Tiwari, "A Brief Introduction to Bhavai | Sahapedia," Sahapedia.org, accessed March 25, 2019, https://www.sahapedia.org/brief-introduction-bhavai.

5. "Bharud is one of those important folk arts of Maharashtra, which is still alive and is going strong even in today's times. After the tamasha, Bharud is next favourite form of folk art in the rural areas, playing an important part of annual fairs. This art form is as educative as it is enjoyable and it is a favourite among the people. It is an important medium to advocate spirituality through drama, elocution and music." "Bhaarud," accessed March 25, 2019, https://web.iiit.ac.in/~sarvesh.ranadeug08/project/bharood/Bhaarud.html.

Case Study: *Cleaner, Healthier, Happier: Using Edutaining Approaches for Shifting Attitudes and Behaviors*

Sonali Khan

India has more than 216 million children under the age of eight who, with the right environment and opportunities, can grow up to be healthy and productive adults. Yet, water, sanitation, and hygiene (WASH)–related diseases impede the survival and growth of those affected by poverty. Unhygienic living conditions, waterborne diseases, and poor sanitation facilities in densely populated slums lead to frequent incidences of diarrheal diseases among children and affect their overall health and well-being.

With support from the Bill and Melinda Gates Foundation, Sesame Workshop India implemented the 'Cleaner, Healthier, Happier' campaign in densely populated slums of Kolkata to provide children access to meaningful sanitation and hygiene messages and to promote safe sanitation practices.

The core idea was to engage and inform children about safe sanitation behaviors through stories, digital games, videos, and print resources. The campaign was conceptualized on the premise that young children can be the change agents for themselves and their communities if the sanitation messages are engaging, child-friendly, and age-appropriate. The power of Sesame Workshop's furry Muppets and media were used to develop key messages for children aged three to eight years old to encourage them to adopt better sanitation practices.

Sesame Workshop India conducted a needs assessment study in Kolkata to identify the existing sanitation-related knowledge and practices and understand the barriers to following safe practices by children. Based on the findings of the study, specific messages and the implementation plan for the pilot phase, which included 500 children and the community were developed. The four core messages developed and tested for appeal and comprehension with children were 'Go to toilet', 'Wear slippers to toilet', 'Wash hands with soap after defecation', and 'Pour water after use'. The pilot study was to determine whether framing the behavior change campaign and its messages as a personal/individual approach that benefits the individual is more effective than presenting them as a collective or 'social' endeavor that benefits the individual (child) and their peers. The objective of this testing was to take the more impactful approach to scale. Based on the results of the pilot, the social or collective approach to behavior change was scaled to reach 50,000 children in 24 Parganas in South Kolkata.

The first task was to get children excited and registered for the campaign. The first two weeks of the campaign were used to create buzz and excitement in the communities by making announcements using megaphones, placing posters and banners at strategic locations, and using branded vegetable carts to showcase songs and short videos to enroll children for the campaign.

The 12-week campaign used a combination of media (video screenings), community engagement with parents, and workshops with children to build their knowledge and influence behaviors. The campaign personified important sanitation-related objects like toilet, water, and soap in the print materials to engage children. Local community barriers such as the lack of soap and availability of water in community toilets were also addressed in the weekly workshops by encouraging children to create soapy threads (threads with single-use pieces of soap strung around them for them to tie as wristbands or necklaces) and tippy tap (homemade water-dispensing containers). A point system was created as an incentive for children who attended workshops and followed safe sanitation behaviors during the campaign.

Based on the learning from the pilot, the scale-up campaign successfully integrated the following components:

1. A social (collective) approach to messaging and behavior change
2. Use of multiple channels like videos, public service announcements (PSAs), print materials, activities, and games for sustained engagement and reinforcement
3. Incentives such as digital games, certificates, and events to motivate children and communities to adopt positive behaviors
4. A specifically designed sanitation Muppet 'Raya' as a role model for children to follow good behaviors

DOI: 10.1201/b23385-28

5. Take-home materials for children to play with their family members and share the key messages

The findings from a qualitative residual study conducted after one year of the campaign indicate that children and caregivers remembered the campaign and its messages, and most children continued to practice safe toilet behaviors. The success of the campaign shows that the early years present a great opportunity to seed long-term habits and behaviors in children. A fun-based approach that engages children and empowers them to become catalysts for real change can successfully promote long-term behavior change.

SECTION IV

HEALTH PROMOTION APPROACHES TO ADDRESS SOCIAL DETERMINANTS AND DISPARITIES

Case Study: *Using Theatre for Health Promotion*

Navsharan Singh

> You don't allow the Dalits to use the farms for their nature's call. You don't allow toilets to be constructed. Where do we go then! So listen, we will queue up in front of your bungalow. We will use the new toilets you have built for yourself, you wait and see.
>
> **Dittu Singh Mazhbi to the village landlord, from the Punjabi play** *The Story of Dittu Singh Mazhbi*

The Census 2011 noted that only 32% of India's rural households had toilets. In 2014, India launched a massive Clean India program to end open defecation and built a large number of household toilets under this program. The available government data claims that by November 2018, 96% of homes had their own toilets. This is up from 38% in October 2014. This is certainly a huge achievement. But while there is plenty of data on toilet construction, there are still questions and an evidence gap about different sections of people having equal access to the same.

In 2015, the WHO/UNICEF Joint Monitoring Programme for Water Supply and Sanitation estimated that 61% of the rural population in India practiced open defecation. The report also placed India as one of the worst performers in the world, strikingly far behind many developing countries including its neighbors Bangladesh, Nepal, Pakistan, and Sri Lanka, which were comparatively ahead of India in meeting the sanitation targets.[1]

Another study revealed widespread rural–urban disparities in terms of housing and toilets. This work, which looked at housing conditions with a special focus on rural India and socially disadvantaged sections, found widespread inequality between rural and urban areas with the proportion of 'good housing' in urban areas far greater than the proportion of 'good housing' in rural areas. Data and evidence also pointed to the caste dimensions of these disparities. The quality of housing data revealed that good housing among the Dalits vis-à-vis others was far worse. The housing survey showed that roughly 50% of Dalits lived in one-room housing units and 64% of these households reported no toilet facility in 2001. This share came down to 54% in 2011. In rural areas, the share of Dalit housing without latrines was 76% in 2011.[2]

What do these statistics and analyses tell us? It shows that rural Dalit households in India are disproportionately disadvantaged when it comes to good housing and access to toilets. But while deprivation and exclusion along the caste lines are evident in data and it is one of the most pervasive inequalities, the mainstream public policy is yet to acknowledge and invest in research and action to tackle caste inequalities concerning access to toilets. However, when access to toilets is mediated by caste, will building more toilets lead to ending open defecation and automatically improving access? When at schools, children are segregated on caste lines, and Dalit children are denied access to school toilets and made to clean the toilets, does the solution to open defecation lie only in building more toilets?[3]

These are India's complex policy challenges. But when it comes to solutions, policymakers typically attribute the widespread open defecation in rural India to poverty, a lack of access to water, and 'backward mindsets'. To date, government sanitation schemes to address open defecation have primarily responded by constructing more toilets and intensifying communications efforts to change the backward mindsets. These 'mindset-changing' communications drives are top-down and often blame the open defecators for being backward.[4] The social and caste barriers and the social, institutional, and policy processes that block access are never mentioned.

This case study is about the significance of the right messaging to bring about change in how access to toilets is understood. *The Story of Dittu Singh Mazhbi* (*Dastan Dittu Singh Mazhbi Di*) is a highly popular Punjabi play about Dalits' struggle in rural Punjab for the right to access toilets. This play gives a different message, one that more visibly and centrally focuses on how power acts as a determinant of access to toilets. It reveals power relations – economic, political, and social – and the injustices that are disproportionately experienced by some groups versus others. The play is about crafting an effective message that neither blames the deprived nor makes an appeal for a change of behavior, but squarely places the right for toilets in the realm of social and political justice. It unpacks the links between access to toilets and caste, and conscientizes the deprived to seek rights and alter the conditions that produce deprivations.

 DOI: 10.1201/b23385-30

Written in 2000 by the well-known Punjabi playwright Gursharan Singh, the play *The Story of Dittu Singh Mazhbi* has been performed hundreds of times in rural Punjab and has changed how open defecation and the need for toilets are understood in rural Punjab. *Dittu Singh Mazhbi* is set in rural Punjab. Dittu, the protagonist, is Mazhbi by caste. Mazhbis are the lowest caste among the Sikhs and though the myth is that Sikhism doesn't practice casteism, Mazhbis are the Sikh untouchables.

Through the life of Dittu, the play uncovers the precarity of the everyday life of a rural Dalit and how it is produced and reproduced through the larger processes of politics and economics. Everyday life also shows the institutional biases and how Dalits' access to resources is perceived as a threat to village hierarchies and power relations.

The backdrop of the play is the changing land and labor relations as a consequence of the farm technology that was introduced in Punjab in the mid-1960s and which goes by the name Green Revolution.[5] The story of the Green Revolution is well known; its early success in Punjab attracted a great deal of attention with the entrepreneurial 'Punjabi Jat-farmer' becoming the icon of this success story. It was only a little later that the strains of technology began to grow on the body politic of the state and a realization came that the increasing gulf between rich and poor farmers, the destruction of the environment, the declining of the water table, and the shrinking access to common resources and work opportunities for Dalit agricultural labor were the consequences of the Green Revolution technology.

Punjab has the highest percentage of Dalits among the states of India, comprising over 31% of the total population. A vast majority of Dalits live in rural areas and they are at the bottom of the social and economic ladder. They are landless (less than 1% percent of rural Dalits own any land), and an overwhelming majority is in agricultural labor. Although they do not own any land, land is a critical resource for the landless laboring families. They need access to land for homestead, fodder, defecation, garbage disposal, tying of cattle, and drying of cow dung cakes, still a major source of household fuel. However, their access and control over common land have changed over the last few decades. Following the Green Revolution and multiple cash crop economies, land has become a highly precious resource: the more land you have, the more you cultivate, and the more profit you make. So over the years, Jat landowners have used their social, political, and economic clout and leveraged caste power to gain control over land and the collective commons. This has resulted in the slipping away of the rights of lower caste landless laborers over commons. The control over land has not only enhanced landowners' returns and power, but it has also increased the vulnerability of the landless, as they are more dependent on landowners for employment, fodder for their cattle, and for the use of fields for relieving themselves.

The Punjab Village Commons Land (Regulation) Act of 1961 allows panchayats to use small parts of village common land for the landless for building houses and other common facilities such as community centers and barat ghars. Common land is also leased to the highest bidder on the condition that a third is reserved for the Dalits and auctioned separately at a lower price. Yet, for years now, Jat landowners have been taking away the common land and subverting the bidding process for the reserved lands in the name of Dalits or through proxy candidates. Whenever Dalits put up resistance and demand that the proxy process be stopped, a 'boycott' is slammed on them by the powerful landowners of the village.

A boycott is a harsh punishment and means that Dalits are stopped from using the field for relieving themselves and from cutting grass for their livestock. The boycott is enforced so severely that if Dalits are seen relieving themselves in the fields or on common lands, they are humiliated and even beaten by the upper caste men. Dalit women, when they go to the fields to gather fodder for cattle, are stalked by the landowners, humiliated, and often sexually harassed. It has not been an uncommon sight in Punjab until very recently to see Dalit men, with women riding pillion on bicycles, going miles away from the village to use an open field for defecating.

The play *The Story of Dittu Singh Mazhbi* is set in this background. Dittu Singh Mazhbi is claiming control over village commons for constructing toilets for Dalits. The upper caste village community claims the rights over village common land to construct a gurudwara, the Sikh temple.

Dittu Singh, an untouchable, is in conversation with the village sarpanch.[6]

Dittu Singh: Tell me Sarpanch. Once it has been decided that the village common land will be used to construct toilets then why are you panicking now!

Sarpanch: This decision had come from the higher authorities. The villagers were not in agreement with it. The previous government had appeased your Dalit community for votes but now the villagers have decided to build a Gurudwara here.

Dittu Singh: Gurudwara?

Sarpanch: Yes Gurudwara. Don't forget that a new government is in place now. Earlier decisions will not be implemented. The foundation stone will be laid by the new MLA. For constructing the Gurudwara, everyone in the region will do voluntary service.

Dittu Singh: Construction through voluntary service?

Sarpanch: Yes, Gurudwaras are constructed this way only. Moreover, this is a historical Gurudwara. Not the sixth but the seventh master of Sikhism set his foot here.

Dittu Singh: How did the seventh master come here?

Sarpanch: The way they come, why do you bother about it?

Dittu Singh: This is your sham. You don't allow the Dalits to use the farms for their nature's call. You don't allow toilets to be constructed. Where do we go then! So listen, we will queue up in front of your bungalow. We will use the new toilets you have built for yourself, you wait and see.

Sarpanch: Is this your threat?

Dittu Singh: You can take it that way!

Sarpanch: With a few votes in hand, these Dalits have the courage now to speak up! We will see you.

(He leaves the stage, and the narrator enters from the other side.)

Narrator: The argument that you just witnessed, you must be thinking that this is just like any other fight between the land owners and Dalits. This fight is bound to happen because for centuries those oppressing would want the oppression to continue. But now this cannot go on like this. If this has to change then it will change, whether it is the Captain or Badal at the head of the government. The play that we are presenting to you now could be the story of any village in Punjab, and the conflict is over latrines.

This play was performed hundreds of times in rural Punjab during the 2000s and is still a popular play. What made it a popular play? Simple, it provided Dalit people the tools to understand why their control over resources slipped away and how they should reclaim it. Dalit discontent and the feeling of powerlessness were lingering in the air, but Dalits needed the tools to understand it. The play came as an agency for education and conscientization, an appropriate communication that challenged the existing top-down understanding, which blamed the victims. The play gave rural Dalit people access and the means to produce, distribute, and share their message.

Following is an excerpt from the final scene.

(Dittu is sitting muttering to himself as the village Sarpanch enters.)

Sarpanch: O Dittu, you are sitting here, and my bungalow is surrounded by your community people and this is all your mischief.

Dittu Singh: No bungalow has been surrounded, just that we have queued up to use your toilet. I had already warned you in advance about it.

Sarpanch: I am the village head and not god who can meet all your needs. I was elected the village head and your community people also voted for me. I spent a lot of money on you people. If now the landlords do not allow you to use their farms for your nature's calls, why should I be held responsible for it? Millions in the country do not have a toilet in their houses, so do they go and surround the house of the elected heads? This is the limit of hooliganism.

Dittu Singh: OK then you tell me, what should landless poor do?

Sarpanch: What can I say, ask the poor people why they are poor? And listen I cannot accept this hooliganism. Tell your community people to stop queuing up in front of my house. I have also informed the police. Then don't blame me for any excesses. Using my toilet ... the cheek of it! The landlords prevent you from using their farms for your nature calls, so does it mean that you go and surround the house of the elected head! Go anywhere and hide behind a shawl for your nature calls.

Dittu Singh: I will tell you one thing. We are starting an operation, "Operation nature's call". Let the police come and round up the Dalit women on their nature's call.

Sarpanch: O Dittu, I know why you are doing all this. But listen, the poor will always remain poor, this is their destiny. Did we tell you to be born in a poor home? You could have been born in a rich man's home. Go ask your fathers and mothers why they give birth to you. I am telling you again that this "Operation nature's call" will not be tolerated.

Dittu Singh: We have queued up and we will only leave when the Sarpanch provides the full account of the money given by the government for constructing the toilets and tell us

why they have not been built. He must promise that the toilets will be made. He must give a written statement and sign it. "Operation nature's call" is continuing.
(Dittu takes out a sheet of paper and gestures Sarpanch to sign. Sarpanch seems shaken and afraid. All freeze. Curtain.)

Not entirely coincidental, nearly a decade and a half since the play was written and first performed, Dalits' claim over village commons is appearing in the news once again and this time the protagonists are Dalit women. In 2016, the Malwa region of Punjab was in the news because Dalit women began mobilizing to claim their rights over the village panchayat land. The mobilization happened in several villages of Punjab over the lack of access to space for defecating and the attack on dignity that it entailed. In the well-known case of the village Matoi, district Sangrur, Punjab, Dalit women were met with heavy resistance and violence when they claimed control over common land through auction. When asked about their agitation they said that they were doing it for their dignity and sexual safety, which is put on the line as they go for open defecation. In bidding for the land, they said, they were not only securing land for their livelihoods but also dignity and sexual safety.[7]

The message of *Dittu Singh Mazhbi* lives on because not only does it uncover the links between toilets and the marginalization of Dalit people in the rural political economy of the state, but it also talks about resistance and mobilization for reclaiming rights and access. The communications message for toilets worked because it was built on Dalits' lived reality and acknowledged the political underpinnings embedded in the inequalities of caste, unequal share in power and prosperity, sexism, and patriarchy, not in norms. Caste inequalities are the result of casteism, not caste norms and stereotypes alone; the intergenerational reproduction of poverty is rooted in institutions and not in mindsets. Prioritizing mindsets as the reason for open defecation depoliticizes the nature of the injustices that disproportionately affect the lower caste. Unless these are confronted head-on, the building of more toilets may not lead to making India clean.

Dittu Singh is talking to himself when his upper caste lady employer enters:

Dittu Singh: Go ahead, build everything for yourself. Don't leave anything for the poor.
Sardarni: What happened Dittu, why are you so angry?
Dittu Singh: Yes I am angry. I have just heard that special schools are being opened in Chandigarh – smart schools which will have arrangements for world class education. Every student will be given a computer. Oh these high class people! They will make 'ideal schools' for their own children. From our children's schools, even the floor mats will be taken away. Bricks will be taken away from the walls. Oh you rulers! This is what your highly paid officers think in terms of governance! Oye pimps, sometime use your brains to think how children of poor people should get good education! How to make studies simple and interesting so that they do not run away from school!
Sardarni: So what kind of education do you want?
Dittu Singh: This is so straight forward. Every child must equally study whether the child is rich or poor. They should have similar schools, similar books, similar school dress. No one should be able to differentiate who is rich and who is a poor kid. France and Canada, I am told, have such a system. But we remain where we were before as if we have sworn not to progress. … And yes, Madam, the Sarpanch has once again put roadblocks to prevent construction of toilets on the village common land.
Sardarni: So why does your representative Shingara Singh not speak up?
Dittu Singh: He has been bought over by the Sarpanch. Every time the bowl licker is up to a new trick.
Sardarni: Bowl licker? Why do you call him bowl licker?
Dittu Singh: His entire character, his thinking is like that of a bowl licker. Whenever upper-caste people drink something, he will lick their cups like a starved person, like a dog licks used utensils for crumbs. It is important to identify and isolate such people.

NOTES

1. 'Progress on Sanitation and Drinking Water—2015 Update and MDG Assessment', cited in Arjun Kumar (2017), 'Households Toilet Facility in Rural India: Socio-Spatial Analysis', *Indian Journal of Human Development*, 11 (1), p. 90.

2. 'Housing Condition in India: With Special Focus on Rural Areas and Socially Disadvantaged Sections', Laurie Baker, Centre for Habitat Studies Vilappilsala, December 2014.

3. See, for instance, Centre for Social Equity & Inclusion (CSEI), Children Movement for Climate Justice (CMCJ), National Dalit Movement for Justice (NDMJ) and Right to Education (RTE) Forum, http://dalitstudies.org.in/wp/wps0101.pdf; https://economictimes.indiatimes.com/news/politics-and-nation/enact-anti-discrimination-in-education-law-ngos-to-government/articleshow/47348153.cms?from=mdr.

4. The communication messages are typically built around an urban *Didi* haranguing the backward rural women on how their practice of open defecation spreads diseases in the family and community, and educates them about the virtues of using a toilet and how it is a happy solution for all problems.

5. The Green Revolution refers to a series of research, development, and technology transfer initiatives, occurring between the 1940s and the late 1960s, that increased agricultural production worldwide, particularly in the developing world, beginning most markedly in the late 1960s. The initiatives, led by Norman Borlaug, the "Father of the Green Revolution" credited with saving over a billion people from starvation, involved the development of high-yielding varieties of cereal grains, expansion of irrigation infrastructure, modernization of management techniques, distribution of hybridized seeds, pesticides, synthetic nitrogen fertilizer, and improved crop varieties developed through the conventional, science-based methods available at the time.

6. The full text of the play in both Gurmukhi and English can be accessed from the Public Archive of Revolutionary Culture Punjab, https://gursharansinghtrust.org/wp-content/uploads/2007/01/Eng-Tr-Story-of-Dittu-Singh-A-Sikh-Dalit.pdf.

7. Aman Sethi, 'The Ekta Club Comes of Age', *Business Standard*, 27 June 2014, https://www.business-standard.com/article/beyond-business/the-ekta-club-comes-of-age-114062701093_1.html.

Case Study

Neeru S. Juneja

Naema, a 16-year-old, was the first one to reach Udyam every day. She ran from school because every day her teacher used to beat her and also ridicule her about her caste. Naema complained to her mother, but her mother didn't have the courage to confront the teacher. One day when Naema's teacher slapped her for no reason, she slapped her back, bit her arm, and ran away from school. That was the end of her education; she was in class 3.

Meenakshi, a very bright girl, was accepted into Pratibha Vikas Vidyalaya, a senior secondary government school for meritorious students, but she had to drop out of school. Because she was intelligent and smart, she had to do everything for her entire family, i.e., going to the ration shop, taking her drunkard father to the hospital, meeting her siblings' teachers, or for that matter anything and everything beyond the four walls of their jhuggi.

After her father died she took up a small job. She was out of school and working. Her dream of becoming a teacher was shattered. Her mother was never happy with her, didn't allow her to take admission to open school, and wanted her to earn more for the family. A bright young girl capable of doing much more was left with no option but to take up petty jobs to make sure that her siblings would not go hungry.

She often questioned, "Didi agar mein ladka hoti tu kya tab bhi mere saath aisa hota?"

Ma'am, would this still happen to me if I was a boy?

DOI: 10.1201/b23385-31

15 Considering the Social, Cultural, and Contextual Factors in Health Promotion

An Anthropological Snapshot

Tulsi Patel

CONTENTS

INTRODUCTION

The historical context of urban planning and the socioeconomic and cultural context of health services reveals a larger picture of public health promotion in practice. The common impression is that health status and facilities are poor in rural and poorer urban pockets in India. Around 70% of India's population is rural and has access to only one-third of the hospital beds; urban dwellers have access to over 65% of the hospital beds (ET 2013). Also, over 64% of healthcare costs in 2013 were met out of pocket, and this was only slightly reduced in 2017–2018 (*The Hindu* 2021). This chapter anthropologically explores the rising medico-technological business of birthing on the one hand and inadequate public health provision and health promoting town planning on the other.

It is well accepted that environmental factors influence people's health status. The mode of development adopted by the world through the exploitation of natural resources and pollution poses huge and unanticipated health risks and complications. The emergence of new viruses has revived both germ and epidemiological theories. Health complications challenge Omran's (1971) theory of epidemiological health transition, whereby societies move from ages of high mortality due to famine and pestilence to somewhat lower mortality from receding pandemics to even more reduced mortality from degenerative and man-made diseases. A different trajectory of disease and demography has emerged with the Ebola, SARS, and COVID-19 pandemics.

A HISTORICAL CONTEXT OF INEQUITY IN HEALTH PROMOTION

The history of medicine in India shows that the rich and ruling elite have had access to better medical services than the poor, and men better than women in colonial India, and the disparity continues. Women in royal families and maharanis expressed health concerns to female Christian missionary doctors, who were deemed not bright enough to be doctors in Britain. They were willing to work in India to provide allopathic care also to ordinary Indian women. It was only much later that hospitals and medical schools that were set up in urban areas started enrolling women to become doctors (Minocha 1996).

INEQUITY IN HEALTHCARE AND SERVICES

The recent Oxfam report (2019) portrays health inequalities between the rich and the poor. Some Indian states have infant mortality rates higher than in sub-Saharan Africa. It laments the government's neglect of public healthcare, meaning the private sector takes over. The very poor have to rely on poor-quality public care or an array of unregulated quacks or take chances with other private providers, often bankrupting themselves in the process. In major cities like Delhi the powerful private corporate hospitals have taken nearly free or heavily subsidized land to build hospitals in lieu of providing a fraction of medical care free of cost to the poor which they rarely do. Many private health corporations have raised government-paid health insurance premiums by three and a half times and threatened to withdraw services if the government fails to comply. Nearly 80% of government insurance payments go to the same hospital corporations. Thus healthcare costs are soaring, pushing millions of households below the poverty line. Private corporation chains are

 DOI: 10.1201/b23385-32

known for being corrupt, charging the government for bogus patients, overcharging, overinvoicing, and prescribing unnecessary interventions and medications (Oxfam, 2019).

BOX 16.1

A highly unethical activity is the removal of young Indian women's uteruses to draw insurance money from the government. Between 2009–2010 and 2014–2015, C-sections, hysterectomies, and other emergency surgeries under NRHM increased by 258% in Bihar and 2215% in Sikkim. The editor of EPW reports on medical overuse, access to surgeries but not basic health care due to increasing insurance health coverage, mushrooming private hospitals, and misuse of government-funded health insurance coverage (EPW 2016: 8).

CITY PLANNING AND INEQUITY IN PUBLIC HEALTHCARE FACILITIES

Urban areas have a higher concentration of medical facilities than rural India. But in cities such facilities are unevenly spread. Since colonial times, Delhi's town planning reveals the in-built health deprivation in Delhi's poorer areas. Ritu Priya (1993) discusses the old urban settlement pattern of Delhi (then Shajahanabad). It had changed since the 1860s to a more open and spread-out pattern. After the mutiny of 1857, more 'sanitized parks' around civil lines areas with ensured sanitation and water supply were created, set up by the Delhi municipal committee. The new capital city, built by Edwin L. Lutyens in 1912, opened more spaces for British officials and other staff outside of the walled city. While the walled city was already congested, heavy in-migration (28% between 1916 and 1926) overcrowded it. The rates of tuberculosis and malaria were alarming. The Delhi Improvement Trust was set up incorporating a public health official. The two parts of the city were strikingly different with more health issues infesting the congested walled city. This pattern of town and city planning was replicated in several cities in India (see Qadeer 2011: 52). The sectoral practice of public health resulted in a decline (Harrison 1994) in death rates in open areas by 80% in the latter half of the 19th and early 20th century.

From 1936 to 1950, the decongestion in Delhi involved the extension of new settlements and the clearing of the slums. But the health of old Delhi residents hardly improved. In the meantime, the deluge of migrants from Punjab, Pakistan, occurred. Housing for the poor was neglected. By 1955 there was a plan for 380,000 houses by 1970. Subsequently, slum resettlement plans were implemented with little thought on public health. These settlements, located near small-scale industries, had roads, electricity, water, drainage, public toilets, parks, shops, schools, dispensaries, and community centers, but lacked potable running water and public transportation, and were overcrowded, making life difficult and exposing residents to diseases. Women were hard-pressed to find exclusive space for bathing and defecating. The lack of sanitation, unclean drains, and waste disposal problems posed constant and major health hazards to the poor. Cyclic occurrences of gastroenteritis, dengue, chikungunya, cholera, and also the Delhi plague in 1994 marked poor public health.

Though Delhi boasts state-of-the-art medical facilities where foreigners seek medical treatment, the poor are overwhelmed by the daily struggle for existence. The poor, in order to save money, prefer to go to self-proclaimed 'medical practitioners' in their localities for quick recovery. They take the pills/powder or colored liquid dispensed by the local practitioners. In contrast, public hospitals mean additional expenses and they are always overflowing with patients, thus visitors are uncertain whether they will be seen by a doctor.

MEDICALIZATION OF CHILDBIRTH

Childbirth in India has long been a family matter. Women gave birth in the privacy of the family home and with assistance from traditional birth attendants. But birthing practices from the West had been brought to hospitals by the turn of the 20th century. Eventually, hospital birthing came to be viewed critically by Western feminists. The birthing business and reproductive technology distanced women's agency as birth givers. For India, arresting population growth was a priority (Patel 2007). By the mid-1960s funding for contraception and birth control was flowing to India. The medicalization of birth in India came through contraception, including abortion technology. The Medical Termination of Pregnancy (MTP) Act was enacted in 1971. The trajectory of the changing terminology of the family planning program kept a tab on the inflow of foreign aid to curtail fertility (Qadeer 2011). In 1992–1993, reducing maternal mortality as well as enhancing maternity care for pregnant women combined with immunization and nutrition strategies were introduced under the Child Survival and Safe Motherhood (CCSM) Programme (GOI 1994).

The National Rural Health Mission (NRHM) has been effective in shifting childbirth from the home to the hospital over the past two decades. Despite a relative increase of 57% in deliveries in institutions during 2005–2008 (Singh et al. 2012) and 80% by 2014 (Joe et al. 2018), there has been only a tiny improvement in the relative perinatal mortality rate (PNMR) of only 2.5%. A United Nations report highlights that India is not training a sufficient number of skilled birth attendants and technical senior managers (Joe et al. 2018). The District Level Health Survey (DHLS) 2007–2008 has revealed substantial gaps in the availability of qualified service providers, equipment, and supplies in primary- and secondary-level healthcare facilities in India. In the Jaipur District, Sharma et al. (2009) acknowledged the popularity of institutional deliveries. Normal deliveries were conducted, but Basic and Comprehensive Emergency Obstetrics Care Centres and Comprehensive Emergency Obstetrics Care Centres were in short supply of very basic and essential drugs such as prenatal antibiotics, misoprostol, and magnesium sulfate. The use of a partograph was absent. Obstetrics care services were poor due to the lack of blood storage units and anesthetists in these centers.

Rising institutional deliveries occur amidst overburdening of facilities, compromising quality of service, and acute shortage of staff at all levels (Sharma et al. 2009). For instance, there were no facilities to keep the mother and baby for 48 hours after delivery owing to infrastructural shortages. Most mothers left as soon as they got the JSY payment. (JSY is a government program under the NRHM that provides cash incentives for institutional deliveries. The birthing woman is paid Rs 1400 [in rural areas] or Rs 1000 [in urban areas], and the Accredited Social Health Activist [ASHA] worker who is the link between the woman and the government is paid Rs 600 [rural] or Rs 400 [urban] for each delivery.)

BOX 15.2

It was found that mothers in some public facilities lay two to a bed with their newborns. During a selection committee meeting interview for a research project on reproductive health, one of the experts, a medical doctor, commented, "You are talking of two to a bed, come with me to my hospital [a public hospital in Delhi], I will show you three to a bed!"

Are birthing complications and maternal mortality unrelated to women's lifelong poor nutritional status? the maternal mortality rate (MMR) among the poor is four times higher than among the well-off (Vishwakarma 1993). Anemia causes bleeding and death, which remains high despite a program to treat it, while the most complex condition, toxemia, has declined (Soman 2004). The Office of the Registrar General (1994), based on existing national data, showed that 65% of all the deaths among women are caused by infectious disease groups and 2.3% are related to childbirth.

LESSONS LEARNED FOR PUBLIC HEALTH AND SUGGESTED MEASURES

We have seen that India's health policy is more favorable to the rich than the poor and men more than women. Women's prior health conditions do matter for maternity outcomes and reproductive health. Urban town planning history in India shows that the poor are discriminated against at the city and health policy planning levels.

Filling vacancies in hospitals is a public health concern. Infrastructure should be enhanced. Taking a life course view of maternal mortality rather than only the reproductive age is needed. Incentivizing facility/hospital births needs a supportive infrastructure for safe delivery and care of the mother. Quality housing is a measure against health risks. City and town planning should be integrated with bettering lifelong nutrition and health for all, including women and the children they bear. More public hospitals, rather than government-financed health insurance, are needed.

REFERENCES

Guha Thakurta, Paranjoy Ed. 2016. Crisis of plenty: The poor in India have access to surgeries but not to basic health care. *Economic and Political Weekly*, 51 (15), 9 April: 8.

Harrison, M. 1994. *Public Health in British India: Anglo-Indian Preventive Medicine 1859-1914.* Cambridge: Cambridge University Press.

Economic Times 2013. Rural India gets access to just 1/3rd of hospital beds. https://m.economic times. com accessed July 3, 2020, https://economictimes.indiatimes.com/industry/healthcare/bio-tech/healthcare/rural-india-gets-access-to-just-1/3rd-of-hospital-beds-study/articleshow/21166646 .cms?from=mdr.

Minocha, A. Women in Modern Medicine and Indian Tradition, in *Social Structure and Change* Shah, A.M., E.A. Ramaswamy and B.S. Baviskar (eds.), New Delhi Sage. 1996: 149–178.

Omran, A.R. 1971. The epidemiological transition. *The Milbank Memorial Fund Quarterly*, 49: 509–538.

Oxfam. 2019. *Public Good or Private Wealth?* Oxfam Report.

Patel, Tulsi. 2007. Female foeticide: Family planning and state society interface in India. In Tulsi Patel (ed), *Sex Selective Abortion in India: Gender, Society and New Reproductive Technologies.* New Delhi: Sage: 316–56.

Priya, Ritu. 1993. Town planning, public health and urban poor: Some explorations from Delhi. *Economic and Political Weekly*, April 24: 824–34.

Qadeer, I. 2011. *Public Health in India: Critical Reflections.* Delhi: Daanish Books.

Singh, S.K., R. Kaur, M. Gupta, R. Kumar. 2012. Impact of national rural health mission on perinatal mortality in rural India. *Indian Pediatrics*, 49: 136–38.

Sharma, M.P. et al. 2009. An assessment of institutional deliveries under JSY at different levels of health care in Jaipur district, Rajasthan. *Indian Journal of Public Health*, 53 (3); 177–82.

Soman, K. 2004. Trends in maternal mortality. *Economic and Political Weekly*, 29 (44): 2859–60.

Vishwakarma, R K. 1993. *Health Status of the Underprivileged.* New Delhi: Radiant and Indian Institute of Public Administration.

16 Addressing Inequities and Vulnerabilities in Health and Development

Can We Close the Gap in a Generation?

Sunanda K. Reddy

CONTENTS

INTRODUCTION

Tackling health inequities is a challenge across the globe that needs to be addressed with a sense of urgency if the Sustainable Development Goals have to be achieved a decade from now.

Public health and population health sciences have a convincing body of evidence showing how social, political, economic, and environmental conditions in people's lives contribute to health inequities and disparities. The impact of deprivation and inequalities in the intersectionality of vulnerabilities in multiple realms affect human development in all its dimensions, including health and well-being.

> The human development approach, rooted in equity and justice, is well established conceptually, yet working toward that development has not adequately translated into the new development paradigm.

While there have been several approaches to promoting health for underserved and marginalized groups, the development and implementation of sustainable strategies for advancing health outcomes for all in the health equity framework deserve greater attention. Health promotion in the context of care and well-being of the vulnerable sections of society requires an understanding of the complex relationship between health and the circumstances in which people live.

As evidence mounts that the most disadvantaged groups in every country are known to have the highest risk of poor health outcomes, the health promotion discourse is moving toward what Sir Michael Marmot referred to as "closing the gap in a generation". Nations must address the mitigation of adverse social circumstances as a means to tackle the intergenerational cycle of health inequities rooted in society and the perpetuating vulnerabilities in the absence of pro-equity interventions at the individual, community, and macro policy levels.

This chapter attempts to look at health inequities through the lens of social justice and a population health equity vision for "leaving no one behind", while advocating for engaging all stakeholders to address the multilevel determinants of health through integrated programs, employing a life course approach.

> *Altering the life course trajectory of risk for poor health in population groups requires an understanding of the factors driving the inequities as well as the changing demands for care over time in an ecological framework.* Addressing the multiple determinants of health at an individual level as well as at the population level in the dynamic model of a complex adaptive system may also call for multiple actors to work harmoniously.

DOI: 10.1201/b23385-33

UNDERSTANDING HEALTH INEQUALITIES, HEALTH INEQUITIES, AND VULNERABILITY

The terms "health inequalities" and "health inequities" are often used interchangeably when describing the health disparities in populations, but the two represent different dimensions of health status experienced by disadvantaged populations.

Health inequality refers to a disparity in health status and/or access to care that characterizes a disproportionate burden of disease or differential utilization of services among individuals or groups within a population.

Health inequity, on the other hand, refers to systematic differences in the opportunities that groups have to achieve optimal health, leading to unfair and avoidable differences in health outcomes.

Equity is set in two dimensions: (i) equality of opportunity and (ii) equality of outcome. *Equality of opportunity* is achieved through procedural justice or 'horizontal equity' in which all are treated the same. *Equality of outcome* is achievable through substantive justice or 'vertical equity' whereby people are treated differently according to the resources, privileges, rights, and fundamental freedoms they might have (or not have).

Equity is a universal concern. For those working with vulnerable groups in the health arena, it is becoming clear that social justice is not possible without strong redistributive policies that can promote communities and public agencies to act coherently in the efforts for gender, racial, ethnic, and social equality for marginalized groups in the intersectionality of vulnerabilities (Figure 16.1).

In advancing the health of underserved populations in low- and middle-income countries, we need to be informed by these concepts and other dimensions of public health in the nuanced discourse that helps us work toward health as a human right as well as a Sustainable Development Goal. All share an association with the social determinants of health (SDH). However, research and services addressing health inequalities or health disparities are targeted toward the gaps in health status experienced by disadvantaged populations. Research and health promotion programs addressing health inequities with a focus on engaging communities and multiple stakeholders to systematically address the structural determinants that produce the social and health inequalities must aim to improve total population health while reducing differences in health outcomes in underserved, underresourced communities.

Vulnerability

Understanding vulnerability must further inform all efforts to improve access to healthcare and impact health outcomes.

Vulnerability may be seen as a state of being in a situation of exposure to the possibility of being harmed physically or emotionally (*Oxford Dictionary*). It is a complex concept with multiple dimensions in different contexts.

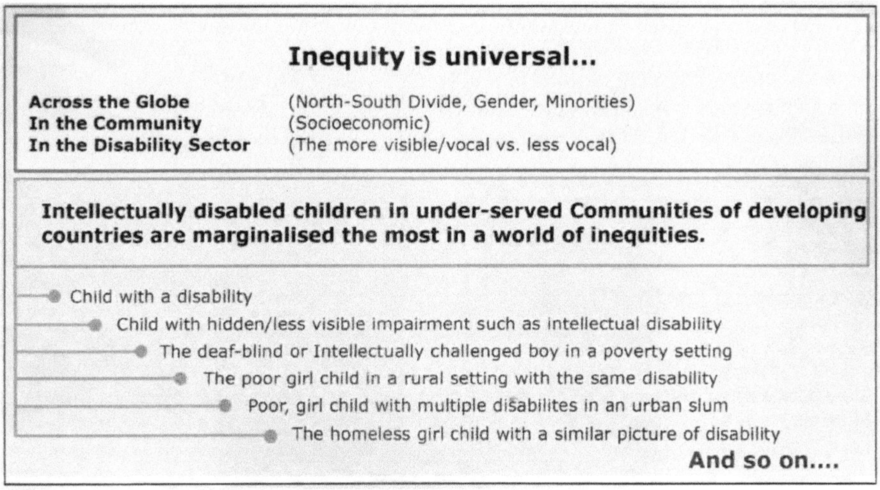

Figure 16.1 Inequity is Universal (From CARENIDHI training modules, 2008.)

Vulnerable groups are many, varying widely in income and social gradients, as well as to the degree to which they experience stigma and neglect. *However, the shared features of discrimination and deprivation of opportunities* to enjoy the fruits of development merit their inclusion in all studies of inclusive and sustainable development.

In the context of multiple vulnerable groups for whom access to healthcare is linked to inequalities in society, it is useful to characterize some groups as more vulnerable due to inherent factors specific to health conditions (e.g., disability) as well as externalities that arise from the intersectionality in cultural contexts and settings. Important among these are children; women; persons with disabilities; sexual minorities; indigenous groups; and people caught in difficult circumstances such as cross-border conflicts, natural disasters, and forced migration. Many of them face deprived opportunities for socioeconomic freedom and fail to reach the optimum potential for human development, of which health is both a determinant as well as an outcome.

BOX 16.1

POINTS TO PONDER

Shabnum is a four-year-old child with cerebral palsy, a neurodevelopmental disability. She lives in an unauthorized urban slum colony with her family. Her parents work for daily wages at a construction site, and her ten-year-old sister takes care of her at home while the parents are at work.

Shabnum has an associated seizure disorder and requires regular medicines. She is also malnourished. In the absence of an integrated program for health and rehabilitation along with nutrition, counseling, immunization, and medicines through primary care, how does this child maintain health?

A hospital visit involves a loss of a day's wages for Shabnum's parents, in addition to incurring the costs of transportation to the hospital for multidisciplinary services. The ten-year-old sibling (who should be in school herself) is the substitute caregiver to deliver health, nutrition, and rehabilitation intervention at home. Is it little wonder then that this child with poor health and multiple vulnerabilities will be lost for follow-up care and will fail to maximize her potential for health and human development.

For someone like Shabnum (see Box 16.1), targeted strategies to address social determinants or only addressing discrimination through policies to promote access to health resources for the marginalized may not suffice. Inequities in child health correlate well with the socioeconomic gradient. The importance of mitigating disparities in socioeconomic circumstances is a definite means to attenuate health inequality.

ON THE PATH TO "HEALTH FOR ALL"

There is a new awareness among nations to invest in population health interventions at the policy and systems levels. There have been good examples of countries addressing inequities through measures of social protection. Many developed countries like the Nordic countries have made it integral to their systems.

BOX 16.2

THE 30 BAHT SCHEME OF THAILAND (2002)

The 30 baht scheme made Thailand the first transition country in Asia to introduce universal health coverage. The aim was to ensure equitable healthcare access to the poorest citizens and provide social protection to the vulnerable sections. Designed by the government and civil society collectively as a part of a comprehensive policy to improve health outcomes, it also had components of income – augmenting schemes for people and institutions delivering the services at minimum cost to citizens. Despite the shortcomings of a shift of services toward curative than preventive, it succeeded in extending coverage of health services to the poor and vulnerable in a focused manner and enabling citizens to recognize healthcare as a right.

This scheme became the forerunner to several social protection schemes in Asia.

Healthcare systems have started partnering with community-based organizations to explore local solutions for implementing service delivery models. One such is when a trained community health worker (CHW) reaches out through a gamut of family-centered services to address girls' and women's health – from discriminatory nutrition to early childbearing and pregnancy complications from anemia and even more ill health from osteoporosis or diabetes in the post-reproductive years with continued discriminatory healthcare. CHW programs in the Indian subcontinent hold much promise, with Accredited Social Health Activists (ASHAs; India) and Swasthya Sebikas (Bangladesh) becoming the backbone for rural health services.

Community-based studies show that contextual factors operate at several levels, notably the environmental level. Integrative population health equity frameworks are looking at the social determinants, community-based, social marketing, health in all policies, and systems approaches integrating community health and clinical practice to reach marginalized groups. Health promotion strategies and targeted health interventions yielding good results in some communities are not able to address on scale the larger political, social, cultural, and economic forces that influence health. The COVID-19 pandemic revealed that global solidarity based on shared values may be as important for equitable population health as shared vulnerabilities for community health. Collaborations widen opportunities for convergence with sectors crucial for determinants of health such as education or the environment can strengthen community health systems to address the determinants of health in the ecological model (Figure 16.2).

When resources are scarce and barriers considerable, working toward the progressive realization of the goal needs innovative approaches. The solution lies, perhaps, in integrating many of the successful approaches and contextualizing interventions at the individual, institutional, and community levels. We must get inclusive in seeking solutions. An integrated paradigm of development

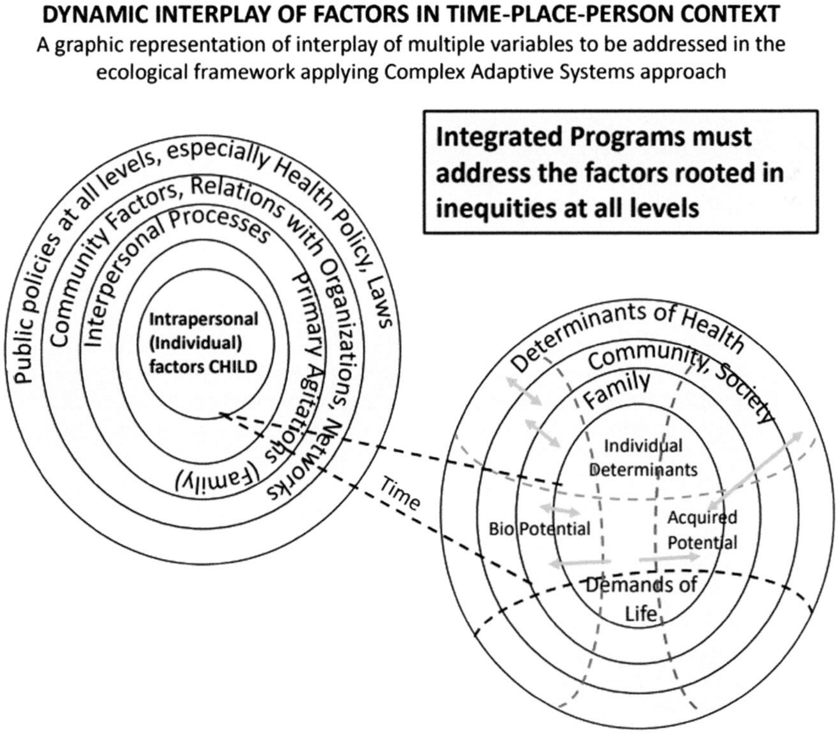

Figure 16.2 Dynamic Interplay of factors in Time-Place-Person context. A graphic representation of interplay of multiple variables to be addressed in the ecological framework applying Complex Adaptive Systems (CAS) approach. *Source:* Formulated by the author.

focused on closing the current gaps in health must involve the participation of vulnerable groups in all community-based inclusive development interventions. This needs to be buttressed by a policy-assistive framework to improve the contexts, behaviors, and experiences at all levels, while recognizing the global influences on health in an ecological model. This translates to a multipronged approach that addresses all components of health as defined by the World Health Organization (WHO), namely, prevention, health promotion, care, rehabilitation, and palliation for all. Health promotion efforts are becoming broad-based with human rights education, legal literacy, welfare economics, and more to ensure a progressive realization of the "health for all" goal. The Indian National HEALTH POLICY, 2017, recognizes this, but the challenges arising from the weak health systems and adverse socioeconomic determinants of health – laid bare and highlighted during the pandemic – make us all too aware that the journey toward universal health coverage can be arduous and with barriers along the way. However, it is a journey that needs to be undertaken, with a good roadmap and preparedness for taking longer, if required, to reach the destination – perhaps not in a generation but in two.

THE WAY FORWARD

> Few disagree with the call for a different path forward, but the nature of that path remains to be determined.
>
> **Jack P. Shonkoff**

If one is speaking of health in the next generations, it has to be built on child health and development today. Addressing inequities begins with understanding the challenges that often occur at birth, continue into early childhood and adolescence, and evolve into the disadvantages an adult faces over the life course.

To begin, *prioritize early childcare and development* (ECD). ECD is an input as well as a tool with the capacity to transform societies. Early childhood is a period when the foundations of lifelong health, learning, and behavior are laid down. We have evidence from neuroscience that the developing brain, with a high degree of neuroplasticity in the early years, is highly responsive to both enriching influences and adverse influences in the environment. Neural epigenetic studies suggest that the long-term effects of early experiences on the developing brain not only compromise the development of children but continue into adulthood and across generations.

Children also represent a vulnerable segment of the population owing to a dependence on adults for nutrition, health, education, and protection from harm. More than 220 million children under five years old are stunted and/or living in extreme poverty. Over 40% of the world's stunted children live in India. As per the Multiple Indicator Cluster Surveys (MICS) using the Early Childhood Development Index measure developed by UNICEF, 37% of children in low- and middle-income countries are showing low levels of cognitive development and socioemotional health. There are inequities in access to health and pre-primary education, with children in the poorest income quintile having less access.

Addressing health inequities in a multidimensional framework requires us to act for mitigation of challenges at birth (including maternal health), invariably continuing into early childhood and adolescence, on to adulthood, and the future generation of children born into the cycle of life with disadvantages. Hence, the need for a life course perspective and a call for "equity from the cradle" as an approach to health in the matrix of sustainable development (Figure 16.3).

Children experience multiple disadvantages at the intersectionality of vulnerabilities and marginalization. For example, children with disabilities in resource-poor community settings, with an added complexity of acculturative stress of migration that families experience in the makeshift neighborhoods, lacking basic amenities for health, in addition to having no access to healthcare and rehabilitation services, are affected the most.

Attention to determinants of disease in populations and mitigation of risks nesting in biological and sociological hierarchies will have to be addressed in a complex, adaptive system framework.

Social determinants of health also have to be seen outside of silos, namely, water, sanitation, air pollution, nutrition, and education, and understood in the dynamic interplay between biology and society, culture and context, and opportunities and capabilities in a time–place–person context for life course approaches to ensure equitable health for future generations.

Integrating actors across sectors for life course approaches (time), with due attention to contexts (social determinants), should be the new paradigm to tackle health inequities rooted in the intergenerational cycle of poverty perpetuation. Collaborations with widened opportunities for convergence with other determinants of health, such as education and the environment, require

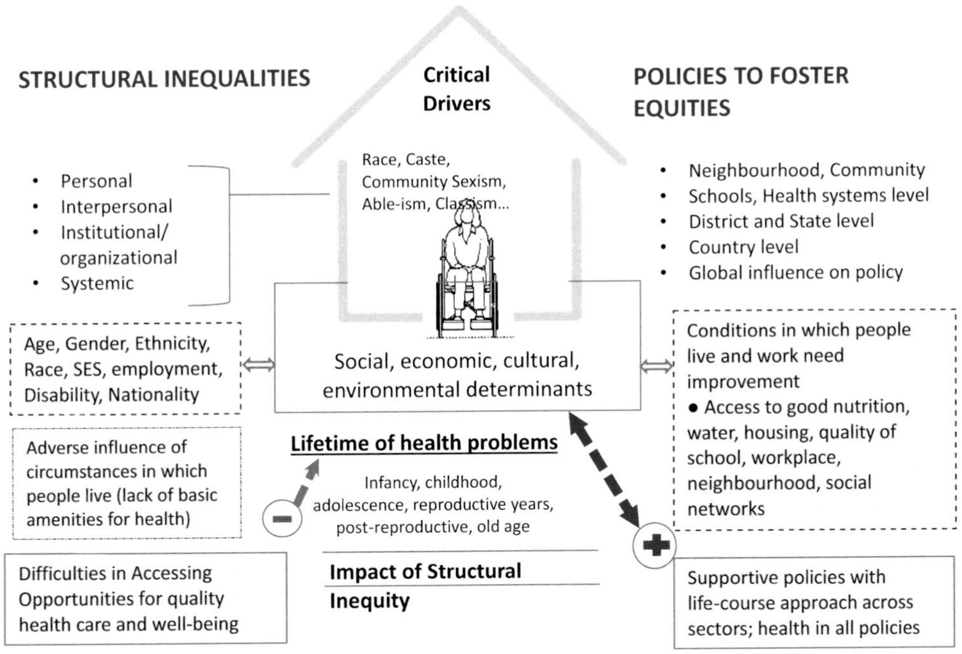

Figure 16.3 Critical drivers of inequalities and facilitators to foster equities. *Source:* conceptualised by Author for this chapter.

adequate allocation of resources to strengthen community health systems in the ecological model. Universal health coverage should be guided by welfare economics and robust health policies for inclusive health programs. Integrative population health networks of community health and clinical practice in a systems approach combined with the health in all policies approach to reach marginalized groups focused on the foundational years of human development may provide the key to a healthy future.

> "Health for all" holds a mirror to sustainable development. It is an achievable goal, provided the political will to tackle health inequities from "womb to tomb" is strong.

REFERENCES

Braveman, P, Gruskin, S. Defining equity in health. *Journal of Epidemiology and Community Health* 2003;57:254–8.

Britto P. Why early childhood development is the foundation for sustainable development. 2015. https://blogs.unicef.org/blog/why-early-childhood-development-is-the-foundation-forsustainable-development/. Accessed August 2019.

CSDH. *Closing the Gap in a Generation: Health Equity Through Action on the Social Determinants of Health. Final Report of the Commission on Social Determinants of Health.* Geneva: World Health Organisation; 2008.

How community-based early childhood programs can impact child development. n.d. Retrieved 22 March 2021, from https://blogs.worldbank.org/education/how-community-based-early-childhood-programs-can-impact-child-development

Mercer R, Hertzman C, Molina H, Vaghri Z. Promoting equity from the start through early child development and health in all policies (ECD-HiAP), *Health in All Policies*. 2013;105. [Internet]. [cited 2021 Feb 10].

Mevawalla Z. The Crucible: adding complexity to the question of social justice in early childhood development. *Contemporary Issues in Early Childhood*. 2013; 14(4):290–299. http://dx.doi.org/10.2304/ciec.2013.14.4.290

Mongkhonvanit PT, Hanvoravongchai P. The impacts of universalization: A case study on Thailand's social protection and universal health coverage. In: Yi I, editor. *Towards Universal Health Care in Emerging Economies*. London: Palgrave Macmillan UK; 2017. p. 119–54.

Sen, A. Capabilities and resources. In: *The Idea of Justice*. Penguin: Penguin Books; 2009, 01/07/2010, 9780141037851.

Shonkoff JP, Garner AS, Committee on Psychosocial Aspects of Child and Family Health, Committee on Early Childhood, Adoption, and Dependent Care, Section on Developmental and Behavioral Pediatrics. The lifelong effects of early childhood adversity and toxic stress. *Pediatrics*. 2012 Jan;129(1):e232–246.

Trinh-Shevrin C, Nadkarni S, Park R, Islam N, Kwon SC. Defining an integrative approach for health promotion and disease prevention: A population health equity framework. *J Health Care Poor Underserved [Internet]*. 2015 May [cited 2021 Feb 10];26(2 Supplement):146–63.

Zubairi A, Rose P, Moriarty K. *Leaving the Youngest Behind*. Research for Equitable Access and Learning (REAL) Centre, Faculty of Education, University of Cambridge; 2019, Theirworld-Leaving-The-Youngest-Behind-2nd-Edition-April-2019.pdf (inee.org).

Case Study

Neeru S. Juneja

> Varsha, still in her teens, was married off way before the stipulated marriageable age. We tried to reason with her parents, but they had a standard answer: "Hamare yaahn aise he hota hai" (This is the norm). Varsha was also happy and excited. She was to get new clothes and jewelry, and have a partner who would love her and share everything. This is what she had learned: a girl has to get married and raise a family. Four months after her wedding, she came back to her parents' place as she was not able to conceive. Her mother-in-law and mother took her to several doctors, but her husband never accompanied her nor was he asked to undergo any tests: "Ladke mein koi nuks nahi hai" (There's nothing wrong with the boy).

Varsha eventually delivered a baby boy, but she was sent back to her mother's place, as other family members felt that she was not good for her husband.

DOI: 10.1201/b23385-34

17 Culture-Sensitive Approaches toward Alleviating Health Disparities for Promoting Health

Venkata Ratnadeep Suri, Mona Duggal, and Neha Dahiya

CONTENTS

INTRODUCTION

Health disparities are defined as those preventable differences between distinct groups of people in the burden of disease, injury, or opportunities to achieve optimal health that are often experienced by socially disadvantaged groups (1). Examples include high incidences of preventable deaths in women of childbearing age in developing countries; high proportions of mortality rates due to communicable diseases; high incidences of malnutrition and related deaths among children under five years of age (2); and certain diseases like depression, osteoporosis, breast cancer, and autoimmune disorders that are more common in women (3).

Traditionally, health promotion interventions aimed at alleviating health disparities have focused primarily on individual and interpersonal factors, which are limited in their ability to yield sustained improvements (4) especially since many are due to the poverty or social determinants of health. However, in recent years, there has been an increasing recognition that health disparities emerge and persist through a complex interaction between socioeconomic, environmental, and system-level factors (4). Some of these factors include gender (male/female), race/ethnicity, socioeconomic status, geography, disability, education level, and immigration and minority status, which affect the symptomatology and outcome of disease (5). Furthermore, health system-related or state-level structural inequalities[1] (systemic and institutional biases in health policies) and institutionalized health policies that segregate based on socioeconomic factors also contribute to health disparities, making factors that contribute to health disparities complex, interdependent, and operational at multiple levels. Therefore, it is important to use rigorously evaluated, evidence-based interventions at multiple levels to address these disparities (4).

CULTURALLY SENSITIVE APPROACH TO HEALTH PROMOTION

In the last decade, there has been an increasing consensus in the field of public health that underscores the importance of developing policies and promotion/communication strategies that are culturally/contextually appropriate, and fundamentally address the structural determinants of health (7). Culturally sensitive health promotion strategies are rooted in the notion that health is determined by a range of sociocultural and structural factors (e.g., access to health, employment), which, in turn, shape individual health behaviors and health inequities (8, 9). Here, culture refers to a wide range of social norms, interactions, values, and perspectives that shape health behaviors within the community (7). Additionally, health-related behaviors become meaningful within specific cultural contexts that are rooted in cultural values, beliefs, and structural factors impacting the daily life experiences of individuals (10). Last, the agency of individuals and communities to adopt healthy behaviors is an outcome that is determined by the complex interaction between structure, human agency, and culture (11). Education plays a huge role and as does socioeconomic status.

Culturally sensitive health promotion strategies focus on (a) understanding the cultural contexts and structural factors that influence individual and community-level risks of health disparities, and how these factors shape health behaviors and outcomes; (b) actively engaging with the community through participatory approaches; and (c) remaining disease-agnostic in their approach,

DOI: 10.1201/b23385-35

and focusing on addressing common risk factors leading to multiple health disparities, thereby altering the context(s) and social structures that shape social and health inequalities (4).

An important question that needs to be asked in this context is: Why is it important to develop culturally sensitive health promotion campaigns? Research in the field of psychology has demonstrated that messages are processed more thoroughly and are more likely to be persuasive if their content is more congruent with or tailored according to audiences' cognitive, emotional, and motivational characteristics. These characteristics, in turn, are strongly dependent on an individual's cultural background, indicating that in order to design effective health promotion campaigns, it is also important to understand the cultural aspects of the audience that shape health behaviors within a social group (12).

For example, the language in which health communication messages are created can have a significant impact on the ability of individuals from a certain group to understand the message and adopt its recommendations. Similarly, a particular group's dietary habits could promote or prevent certain diseases. The preceding two examples may be treated as direct effects. On the other hand, though cultural attributes such as collectivism are not directly health-related, they might also influence health behaviors and outcomes. For example, collectivist values such as social conformity and reciprocity are positively associated with the adoption of health behaviors and building community capacity (13), and a reduction in infectious diseases and zoonotic diseases (14). A collectivist culture values the needs of the community over individualistic needs and working together to create harmony, and group cohesion is extremely valued. Social conformity refers to the adoption of specific behaviors by individuals to conform to social expectations, often to fit into a group, or in support of a common social cause or value(s). Reciprocity refers to the adoption of a specific behavior by individuals in response to others adopting the same behavior. Social conformity and reciprocity are related in that the pressure to conform or seeing others conform to these social norms results in the individuals reciprocating by adopting the same behavior, either due to social pressure or for the common good of the society. For example, in the fight against COVID-19 in India, a telephonic public health campaign focusing on educating people about maintaining social distancing and wearing masks was framed in terms of socially responsible behavior to protect oneself and also not infect others, and as a responsibility toward society (reciprocity) as a means of fighting COVID-19 together as a community and as a nation (community capacity building) (15).

Furthermore, research also shows that the congruency between the message design and content, and the mechanism of delivery, in turn, will enhance the persuasiveness of the message. Deeper processing of information, in turn, leads to greater engagement with the content within the message and is likely to enhance compliance with the prescribed health behaviors (16).

STRATEGIES FOR CREATING CULTURALLY SENSITIVE HEALTH PROMOTION CAMPAIGNS

In recent years, several public health practitioners and health communication scholars have provided many useful conceptual frameworks for developing culturally appropriate health promotion campaigns. Of these, the cultural sensitivity approach (17) recognizes two important dimensions of culture that need to be considered when developing health promotion strategies: surface structure and deep structure. Though, in theory, these are considered as two distinct sets of cultural attributes, in reality, most health promotion campaigns that adopt a culturally sensitive approach incorporate both surface-level and deep structural cultural attributes into their campaigns. Surface structure approaches or peripheral strategies (18) refer to matching health messages to observable or "superficial" characteristics of the intended population. These strategies include, but are not limited to, using colors, images, fonts, pictures of group members, or declarative titles that explicitly portray relevance to the group; using local language or dialect to develop health communication messages or promotion strategies (linguistic strategies); choosing specific channels of communication that help reach out to community members directly (e.g., community media, social networks); varying the modes of communication (e.g., street plays, puppet shows, or other folk art forms); and using of community institutions for outreach (e.g., through places of workshops, local schools, and community centers). Furthermore, to enhance the perceived relevance of a health issue for a particular group, health educators may also provide medical evidence of its impact on that particular group (evidential strategies) (18). It follows that surface structure strategies refer to the extent to which health promotion campaigns resonate well with the target population in terms of where they are, and how well they fit within the realm of their day-to-day cultural experiences. For example, the Revised National Tuberculosis Control Programme[2] in India has now adopted strategic culture-specific health communication strategies to reach out to wider audiences. It addresses surface-level cultural attributes by using the local language and dialects, and appropriate channels of communication such as regional folk media, puppet shows, street theater, and rallies.

Deep structural attributes (or sociocultural strategies) are more complicated, have only received greater attention in recent years, and account for a wide range of environmental and psychological forces in addition to surface-level attributes that may impact health. It involves understanding how sociodemographic and ethnic populations differ in terms of their core cultural values, and a range of social, environmental, and historical factors. This is also accompanied by identifying social structures in which community members are embedded, which may limit access to specific health resources and services, and influence specific health behaviors and outcomes. Here, social structures refer to rules, regulations, and norms of governance and organizing that either enable or constrain access to a range of health resources for a particular group of people. Deep structural approaches or sociocultural strategies often emphasize a participatory approach and draw upon the experiential knowledge of the community members (19, 20). Figure 17.1 illustrates the various stages and important factors of a culturally sensitive health promotion campaign.

In recent years, community-based participatory approaches (based on structural perspectives) to reducing health disparities have gained traction. There are two variations of such participatory approaches that have received wider recognition, owing to the number of successfully implemented projects based on these models. These are community-based participatory research (CBPR) (21, 22) and the culture-centered approach (CCA) to health (10). Both CBPR and CCA emphasize the participation of community members in defining the community's health problems and collaboratively exploring a range of feasible solutions to address these challenges. The CCA differs from CBPR in terms of the extent of participation and the role of the community members in the decision-making process. In CBPR, community members and health experts interact to identify the problems and develop solutions, often within the parameters set up by the experts or funding agencies. Furthermore, CBPR approaches are often used to facilitate the adoption of health interventions at the community level (21). In contrast, in the CCA process, both the definition of the problem as well as the solution to the problem originate from within the community and are grounded in the ideas and perspectives developed by community members through discussions and dialogue (20).

The central tenet of such an approach is to integrate the diverse voices from these communities to identify the structural inequities and conditions that shape their health experiences, from the viewpoint of the community stakeholders. The idea is to help the community define its health problems as well as develop solutions to address them. Table 17.1 outlines the similarities and differences between the CBPR and CCA approaches to health communication and health promotion.

CULTURE-CENTERED APPROACH TO HEALTH PROMOTION

In recent years, there has been an increasing realization within the public health community that apart from individual-level factors related to behavioral change, community-level and structural factors also play an important role in the incidence, spread, and possible control of HIV/AIDS (26, 27). For example, the Sexually Transmitted Diseases (STD)/HIV Intervention Project (SHIP) that was implemented in Sonagachi, Calcutta, West Bengal, is considered one of the most successful, longest-running health promotion campaigns in India that targeted the health problem at multiple levels. It focused on addressing several community-level and structural factors to increase the uptake of condom usage among sex workers. It brought down the spread of HIV and AIDS within this community using the CCA approach. The SHIP program consisted of the following key components that are rooted in a CCA: addressing the structural constraints that shape health outcomes (20), problem framing (prostitution as a stigmatized profession vs. sex work as an economic activity), political advocacy, multiple levels of interventions, and sustainability (26). Table 17.2 provides more information about the various components, along with specific examples from the SHIP program that represent each of these concepts (26). The program has received considerable global visibility and has been replicated in a number of countries around the world. As a result of this program, the rate of HIV infection among sex workers significantly reduced and is about 11% (29). Furthermore, as per the data, condom use was consistently on the rise during the duration of the program's implementation – from 3% in 1992 to 90% in 1999 (30).

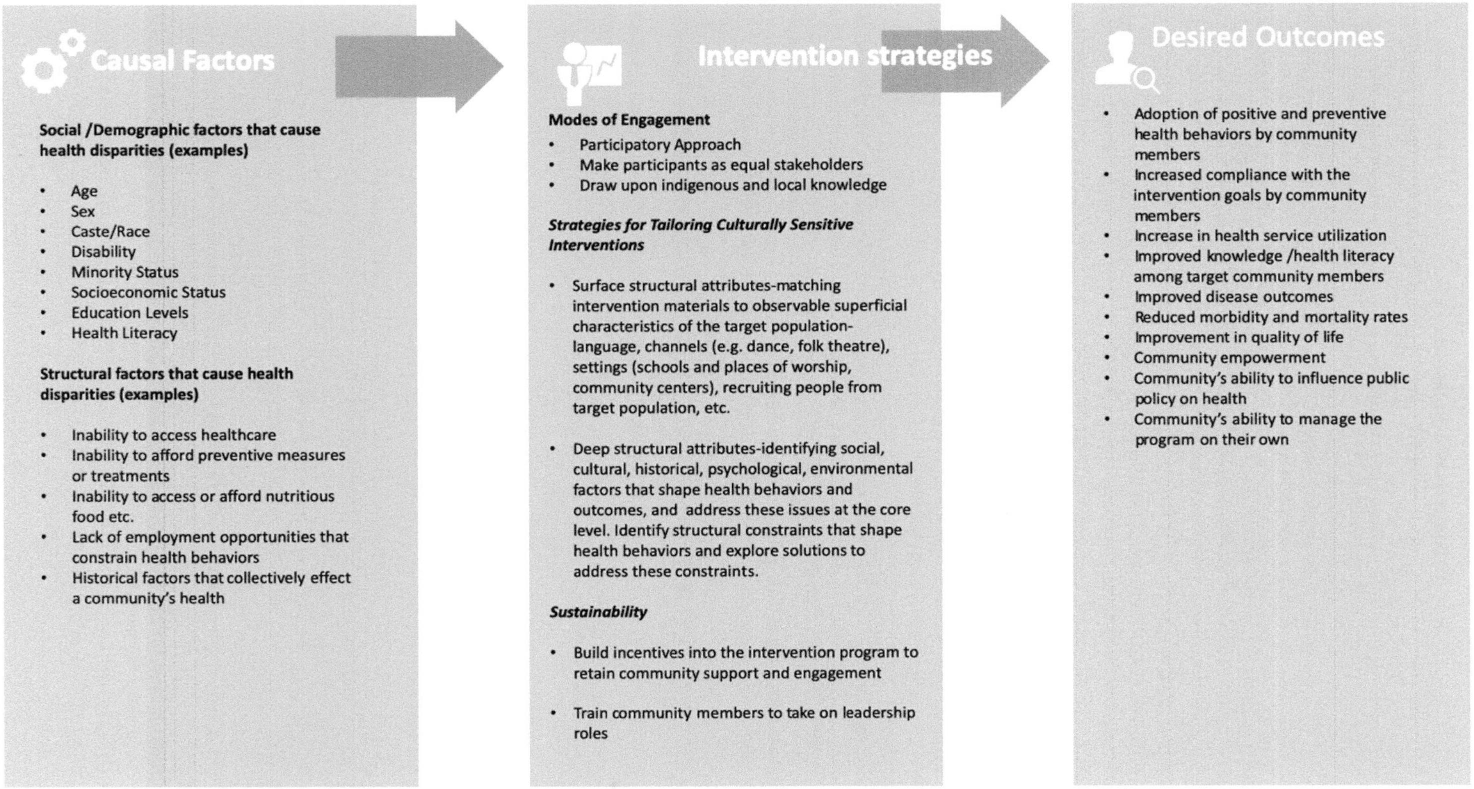
Causal Factors
Social /Demographic factors that cause health disparities (examples)
Age
Sex
Caste/Race
Disability
Minority Status
Socioeconomic Status
Education Levels
Health Literacy
Structural factors that cause health disparities (examples)
Inability to access healthcare
Inability to afford preventive measures or treatments
Inability to access or afford nutritious food etc.
Lack of employment opportunities that constrain health behaviors
Historical factors that collectively effect a community's health
Intervention strategies
Modes of Engagement
Participatory Approach
Make participants as equal stakeholders
Draw upon indigenous and local knowledge
Strategies for Tailoring Culturally Sensitive Interventions
Surface structural attributes-matching intervention materials to observable superficial characteristics of the target population-language, channels (e.g. dance, folk theatre), settings (schools and places of worship, community centers), recruiting people from target population, etc.
Deep structural attributes-identifying social, cultural, historical, psychological, environmental factors that shape health behaviors and outcomes, and address these issues at the core level. Identify structural constraints that shape health behaviors and explore solutions to address these constraints.
Sustainability
Build incentives into the intervention program to retain community support and engagement
Train community members to take on leadership roles
Desired Outcomes
Adoption of positive and preventive health behaviors by community members
Increased compliance with the intervention goals by community members
Increase in health service utilization
Improved knowledge /health literacy among target community members
Improved disease outcomes
Reduced morbidity and mortality rates
Improvement in quality of life
Community empowerment
Community's ability to influence public policy on health
Community's ability to manage the program on their own

Figure 17.1 Culturally sensitive health promotion process.

Table 17.1: Comparison of Community-Based Participatory Research (CBPR) and Culture-Centered Approach (CCA)

Factor	Community-Based Participatory Research (CBPR)	Culture-Centered Approach (CCA)
1. Nature of collaboration	I. Community–academia partnerships. II. Select community members serve as representatives of the community. III. Emphasis is on creating collaborative relationships with community members to implement health promotion programs. IV. Less emphasis on public advocacy and influencing policy changes at the local and global levels.	I. Community–academia partnerships. II. Community members generally serve as change agents in implementing the project by creating cohesive groups that drive social change. III. Emphasis is on creating collaborative partnerships. IV. Creation of communication forums for community members to interact and voice their opinions, and to connect to the dominant actors in the mainstream, power structures, and key decision-makers within the society (e.g., local governments, nonprofit organizations, policymakers, and other key advocacy groups).
2. Methodological approaches used to engage with the community/community members	I. Focus groups. II. Participant observation. III. Interviews with key stakeholders.	I. Focus groups. II. Participant observation. III. Interviews with key stakeholders.
3. Method of defining a social problem 4. Generating solutions to resolve the problems 5. Evaluation of outcomes	I. Generally, the problem is defined by the funding agency/academic partner. II. Solutions are generally based on knowledge transfer by the academic partner/funding agency. III. Project outcome evaluations generally drive the project objectives. IV. Evaluation is generally driven by epistemic objectivity and often conducted using survey methods, etc.	I. Community members identify the health challenges faced by the community. II. Community members define the goals and objectives of the health promotion campaign. III. Community members identify the structural factors that constrain the adoption of desired health behaviors. IV. Community members develop strategies to dismantle these structural constraints. V. Evaluation goals are generally decided in terms of what is important for both community members as well as the collaborating academics and agencies.
6. Sustainability	Long-time sustainability is less emphasized as opposed to meeting the goals and objectives outlined by the program on a short-term basis.	Significant emphasis on creating mechanisms and infrastructures for the long-term sustainability of the interventions.
7. Reflexivity–research–community power relationships	Less emphasis is placed on interrogating the power relationships between the researcher and the community members.	Significant emphasis is placed on constantly interrogating the power relationships between the researcher and the community to ensure that the voices of the community are not ignored.

Sources: Table prepared from information obtained from several scholarly works (20, 22, 23–25).

Table 17.2: Key Components of Sonagachi's Sexually Transmitted Diseases (STD)/HIV Intervention Project (SHIP)

Key Component	Description	Outcomes
1. Recognizing structural constraints that shape health outcomes and exploring solutions from within the community	Participatory community meetings and discussions helped identify several structural constraints that shape health behaviors and outcomes among sex workers.	Several solutions to address the structural barriers to healthcare emerged from within the community were integrated into the intervention program. Example of barriers: Refusing sexual intercourse without a condom can turn away many clients, resulting in economic losses to sex workers. Community developed solution: Establish a microcredit lending system that helps sex workers who are facing economic setbacks to offset economic losses due to losing clients (28).
2. Problem framing	Reframing prostitution (a morally stigmatized occupation) into sex work (an economic activity on par with other forms of livelihood).	• Role of sex workers in the community's economy was recognized. • Prevention of HIV and AIDS was seen as a hazard to the local economy, and its elimination was recognized as a necessary step to save the local economy. • Enforcing condom use and safe sex practices for sex work were seen as a means of continuing the status quo in maintaining the economic interests of various stakeholders in the sex trade. • Various economic stakeholders in the sex work industry, including landowners (who rent rooms to sex workers), pimps, regular clients (a primary source of income for some of the sex workers), local organized crime, police (who receive bribes), and local political agents (who need votes during elections) started supporting the program.
3. Political advocacy	Sex workers from SHIP established the Durbar Mahila Samnwaya Committee (DMSC) forum to advocate for recognizing sex work as a legitimate economic activity, a healthy and safe work environment, access to education for themselves and children, freedom of movement, right to voice their opinions, and access to healthcare facilities.	• Sex worker's rights were well recognized and have gained legitimacy at various political forums. • Today, DMSC is recognized as a sex worker advocacy group that is well connected with several advocacy groups, and AIDS and sex worker conferences from around the world.
4. Multiple levels of intervention	• Group-level intervention: Older sex workers were recruited as "peer outreach workers" who were affiliated with the local health clinic. Peer outreach workers provided a variety of medical services and safe sex education to sex workers. • Individual-level Intervention: Peer outreach workers educated illiterate sex workers about HIV and safe sex methods. • Outreach workers became role models for other sex workers. • Community-level intervention: Various economic stakeholders in the sex work industry were involved in the program.	• The program received greater acceptance among sex workers due to the involvement of peer outreach workers. • Sex workers were willing to get tested. • Sex workers were willing to use condoms and other safe sex practices. • There was a significant increase in condom usage and other HIV prevention steps by sex workers.
5. Sustainability	• The program and its objectives evolved incrementally over time in concert with available resources. • Continuous networking with donors, media, and other nongovernmental organizations worldwide gave it visibility and more funding. • Several economic and social components were built into the program for its long-term sustainability, e.g., sale of condoms by sex workers and a microcredit system of lending. • Power relationships: Over time, many sex workers were increasingly promoted to positions of authority within the program and worked in full partnership with professional staff.	• Incremental success in each stage of the project, in turn, promoted the program's visibility and prestige, thus attracting additional funding. • Networking further increased visibility and attracted donor funding. • Economic incentives such as condom sales provided a means of additional income within the program. It instilled a sense of efficacy and competence among the sellers. • The microcredit system helped offset economic losses for sex workers who adopted safe sex practices at the cost of losing clients. • The microcredit system helped sex workers to start small businesses and other means of income that sustained their participation in the program. • Establishment of the DMSC forum, from which members are drawn from within the local community. This ensured that community members play an important role in sustaining the project. The DMSC represented sex workers' rights and issues at various global and local venues, and with the local government and leadership. • The involvement of sex workers in positions of power, including membership in the DMSC, shifted the ownership to the community, which contributed to the project's long-term sustainability.

Sources: Table prepared from information obtained from several scholarly works (25, 26).

BOX 17.1 KEY TAKEAWAYS

1. Health is an outcome of a complex interaction between structure, human agency, and cultural factors
2. Both surface structure and deep structure cultural attributes play an important role in people's ability to relate to and comprehend health information, and to act upon this information in order to address their health issues.
3. Identifying and addressing structural factors that shape people's ability or inability to adopt healthy behaviours is key to successfully addressing health disparities in different communities.
4. Culturally sensitive health promotion campaigns must find ways to inculcate culture-specific practices to make these campaigns effective in dealing with health disparities.
5. Culturally sensitive health campaigns are likely to be successful if community members become equal stakeholders, as this will empower them to take responsibility and build the community's capacity to address health inequities.

CONCLUSION

Health and health disparities are the outcome of a complex interaction between individual-level factors, and a range of social, economic, environmental, and policy-level factors that determine the health status of individuals and communities. In recent years, there has been a push toward developing health promotion strategies and policies to address both individual- and structural-level factors that shape health disparities. In this chapter, we introduced the idea of culturally sensitized health promotion strategies as a viable means to address multiple factors that shape health disparities. Using the cultural sensitivity framework (17), we discussed two important dimensions of cultural attributes that need to be considered when developing health promotion strategies – surface structure attributes and deep structure attributes – and we provided several examples of both of these cultural attributes. With health promotion strategies that imbibe both surface structural attributes gaining importance in the domain of public health, we briefly discussed two distinct methods of health promotion that are based on deep structural approaches.

Using several examples from health promotion projects that incorporated and addressed both surface and deep structure cultural attributes, we identified several cultural dimensions that can be considered when designing a health promotion campaign (26).

Although every social context is different, some of the theoretical ideas and their instantiations in the form of examples that we provided will hopefully serve as a heuristic framework to identify a range of cultural attributes that can be considered when designing culturally sensitive health promotion campaigns aimed at addressing the core factors that shape a range of health disparities.

ACKNOWLEDGMENTS

This chapter greatly benefited from editorial comments from Dr. Akanksha Bapna.

NOTES

1. For example, the "Ayushman Bharat Yojana," a national health insurance scheme being implemented in India, provides coverage in secondary and tertiary hospitals to only 40% of the poor and vulnerable population of the country. Additionally, participating states are compelled to contribute to the insurance scheme, which in turn diverts funds that are to be used for revamping the healthcare system in participating states, further contributing to disparities in access to healthcare in these states (6).

2. Bhavan N., National Strategic Plan for Tuberculosis Elimination 2017–2025, Ministry of Health and Family Welfare, 2017;109.

REFERENCES

1. Braveman P. What are health disparities and health equity? We need to be clear. *Public Health Rep.* 2014;129(Suppl 2):5–8.

2. Menon GR, Singh L, Sharma P, Yadav P, Sharma S, Kalaskar S, et al. National burden estimates of healthy life lost in India, 2017: An analysis using direct mortality data and indirect disability data. *Lancet Glob Health*. 2019;7(12):e1675–84.

3. What health issues or conditions affect women differently than men? [Internet]. https://www.nichd.nih.gov/. 2020 [cited 2020 Jul 27]. Available from: https://www.nichd.nih.gov/health/topics/womenshealth/conditioninfo/howconditionsaffect

4. Structural interventions to reduce and eliminate health disparities. *AJPH*. 109(S1) [Internet]. [cited 2020 Jul 27]. Available from: https://ajph.aphapublications.org/doi/10.2105/AJPH.2018.304844

5. Cowling K, Dandona R, Dandona L. Social determinants of health in India: Progress and inequities across states. *Int J Equity Health*. 2014;13(1):1–12.

6. Paul V. Ayushman Bharat Pradhan Mantri Jan Arogya Yojana (AB PMJAY): Hope for millions and exciting new prospects for neuro-healthcare. *Neurol India*. 2019;67(5):1186.

7. Airhihenbuwa CO, Ford CL, Iwelunmor JI. Why culture matters in health interventions: Lessons from HIV/AIDS stigma and NCDs. *Health Educ Behav*. 2014;41(1):78–84.

8. Marmot M. Social determinants of health inequalities. *Lancet*. 2005;365(9464):1099–104.

9. Napier AD, Ancarno C, Butler B, Calabrese J, Chater A, Chatterjee H, et al. Culture and health. *Lancet*. 2014;384(9954):1607–39.

10. Dutta MJ. Communicating health: A culture-centered approach. *Polity*. 2008 Feb 4.

11. Dutta MJ. Cultural context, structural determinants, and global health inequities: The role of communication. *Front Commun*. 2016;1:5.

12. Airhihenbuwa CO, Makoni S, Iwelunmor J, Munodawafa D. Sociocultural infrastructure: Communicating identity and health in Africa. *Journal of Health Communication* 2014 Jan 1;19(1):1–5.

13. Betsch C, Böhm R, Airhihenbuwa CO, Butler R, Chapman GB, Haase N, et al. Improving medical decision making and health promotion through culture-sensitive health communication: An agenda for science and practice. *Med Decis Making*. 2016;36(7):811–33.

14. Morand S, Walther BA. Individualistic values are related to an increase in the outbreaks of infectious diseases and zoonotic diseases. *Sci Rep*. 2018;8(1):1–9.

15. Abbott S, Freeth D. Social capital and health: Starting to make sense of the role of generalized trust and reciprocity. *J Health Psychol*. 2008;13(7):874–83.

16. Pasick RJ, D'onofrio CN, Otero-Sabogal R. Similarities and differences across cultures: Questions to inform a third generation for health promotion research. *Health Educ Q*. 1996;23(1_suppl):142–61.

17. Resnicow K, Baranowski T, Ahluwalia J, Braithwaite R. Cultural sensitivity in public health: Defined and demystified. *Ethn Dis*. 1998;9(1):10–21.

18. Kreuter MW, Lukwago SN, Bucholtz DC, Clark EM, Sanders-Thompson V. Achieving cultural appropriateness in health promotion programs: Targeted and tailored approaches. *Health Educ Behav*. 2003;30(2):133–46.

19. Airhihenbuwa CO, Liburd L. Eliminating health disparities in the African American population: The interface of culture, gender, and power. *Health Educ Behav*. 2006;33(4):488–501.

20. Dutta MJ. Culture-centered approach in addressing health disparities: Communication infrastructures for subaltern voices. *Commun Methods Meas.* 2018;12(4):239–259.

21. Minkler M, Wallerstein N. *Community-Based Participatory Research for Health: From Process to Outcomes.* John Wiley & Sons; 2011.

22. Israel BA, Eng E, Schulz AJ, Parker EA. *Methods for Community-Based Participatory Research for Health.* John Wiley & Sons; 2012.

23. Hamilton KC, Henderson Mitchell RJ, Workman R, Peoples EA, Higginbotham JC. Using a community-based participatory research approach to implement a health fair for children. *J Health Commun.* 2017;22(4):319–26.

24. Basu A, Dutta MJ. Sex workers and HIV/AIDS: Analyzing participatory culture-centered health communication strategies. *Hum Commun Res.* 2009;35(1):86–114.

25. Basu A, Dutta MJ. Participatory change in a campaign led by sex workers: Connecting resistance to action-oriented agency. *Qual Health Res.* 2008;18(1):106–19.

26. Jana S, Basu I, Rotheram-Borus MJ, Newman PA. The Sonagachi Project: A sustainable community intervention program. *AIDS Educ Prev.* 2004;16(5):405–14.

27. Kelly JA. Community-level interventions are needed to prevent new HIV infections. *Am J Public Health.* 1999;89(3):299–301.

28. Baker EA, Motton FL. Creating understanding and action through group dialogue. *Methods Community-Based Particip Res Health.* 2005 Aug 19;307–25.

29. Joint United Nations Programme on HIV/AIDS, World Health Organization. *Epidemiological Fact Sheets on HIV/AIDS and Sexually Transmitted Infections.* 2004.

30. National AIDS Control Organization (India). *National Aids Prevention and Control Policy.* National AIDS Control Organisation, Ministry of Health & Family Welfare; 2001.

Index

Q

R

S

T

U

V

W